S0-BSV-102

THE *NEW* AEROBICS

THE
NEW
AEROBICS

BY

KENNETH H. COOPER,
M.D., M.P.H.

published by

M. EVANS AND COMPANY, INC.,
New York

Withdrawn

DEDICATION

To my wife, MILLIE, *who has become a tireless co-worker, an unwavering supporter, and a beautiful example of the benefits of regular exercise—and to my young daughter,* BERKLEY, *who has learned to live so often and so much without Daddy.*

90222

Copyright © 1970 by Kenneth H. Cooper
All rights reserved under International and
Pan-American Copyright Conventions
Library of Congress Catalog Card Number 78-88699
ISBN 0–87131–028–7
Manufactured in the United States of America

15 14 13 12 11 10 9 8 7

Author's Preface

WHEN I INTRODUCED aerobics as a new concept of exercise, my chief aim was to counteract the problems of lethargy and inactivity which are so widely prevalent in our American population. Therefore, my first book was mainly a motivational book, but also it was an attempt to encourage people to examine more closely the benefits to be gained from regular exercise. The wide public acceptance of *Aerobics* indicates that these objectives have been at least partially achieved.

The present volume serves a different purpose. As a result of the comments from people in all walks of life and the accumulation of vast amounts of new data, it has been possible to prepare a book which discusses in great detail the specific requirements for safely and effectively entering an age-adjusted exercise program. I tend to classify this book more of an "Aerobics Handbook" or an "Aerobics Guidelines" than a new concept of exercise. For this reason, I hope that the faithful follower of "Aerobics" as well as the unconditioned beginner will find this new version of aerobics both interesting and challenging. Because of the expanded range of exercise options, the adjustment for age, and the comprehensive data tables, I also hope that physical educators and medical personnel concerned with exercise will find this book useful in supervising physical conditioning programs.

Whether this book is used as an individual exercise guide or as a professional reference work, it is my profound hope as a physician that it will serve its readers as a key to health and well-being.

KENNETH H. COOPER, M.D.

San Antonio, Texas

ACKNOWLEDGEMENTS

Many people were involved in the preparation of this book but I am especially indebted to Dr. Jere H. Mitchell, professor of physiology and associate professor, Department of Medicine, Southwestern Medical School, Dallas, Texas, for his review and critique and to Mr. Hans Fantel for his invaluable assistance in the preparation of the manuscript. Colonel Clifford Raisor helped immensely in expediting the administrative review of this book and his comments and advice were a continual source of encouragement.

Contents

1: The Impact of Aerobics

I RECEIVED A letter recently from an elderly gentleman who wrote:

Dear Dr. Cooper:
I want to take this opportunity to thank you for the Aerobics conditioning program. I have followed the program faithfully for over nine months. During the past six months, I have been averaging at least 30 points per week entirely by walking. I sleep better, feel better, and have gone through the winter without any medical problems for the first time in years—and I am anxiously awaiting my 94th year.

Appreciatively,

This is one example of the thousands of letters I have received from men and women, of all ages, and from all over the world. Many are letters of appreciation. Others ask questions. But nearly all document the beneficial effect aerobics has had on their lives. It has been impossible to respond to all of these letters, so I hope that this book will in some way serve as a means of communicating with dedicated aerobics fans everywhere. Perhaps it will inspire others to began an aerobics program. But my most earnest hope is that the wisdom gained from testing and training tens of thousands of men and women can be imparted to people everywhere who are still seeking healthier, more productive and more effective lives.

Today, the official physical fitness program of the United States Air Force is based on aerobics, with roughly 800,000 members of the Air Force participating. Several foreign military organizations are considering adopting it as their official conditioning program. What's more, aerobics is no longer exclusive to the military. Countless people in every walk of life have found aerobics a workable way to achieve new levels of physical competence and personal well-being. Professional athletic teams have found it to be an excellent way to maintain a high level of fitness during the off season. Many colleges and universities throughout the country have adopted aerobics as a part of their physical education program. All have shown interest in the program because it is the first scientific attempt to validate and quantify the effect of exercise~and to answer the intriguing questions of what kind, how often, and how much.

The age range of the participants in this program has also been remarkable. I was surprised to discover that a large proportion of aerobics fans—women as well as men— are in the 40–60 age bracket. The men in this age group say that they took up aerobics as a type of life insurance. And the women admit just as frankly that they consider aerobics a good way to keep their figures as well as their health.

A middle-aged woman writes:

After raising a family of four children, I could once again concentrate on regaining a youthful figure. I tried dieting but always seemed to lose weight where I didn't want to. When I combined a mild dietary restriction program with aerobics, I lost weight and inches in desirable places—hips, thighs and waist. I dropped three dress sizes and my husband says I look ten years younger! Aerobics has completely changed my life.

I have also learned that these [middle-aged men and women respond well to training programs but that their approach must be less vigorous and more prolonged. Consequently, you will notice that there are four age-adjusted conditioning programs in the center of this book. In addition, physical fitness categories have also been age-adjusted. And for the older person, there has been more emphasis placed on achieving 30 points per week as contrasted to meeting the requirement of a physical fitness test. As a result, the program is now more adaptable and easier to accomplish by men and women of all ages.

The widespread interest in exercise has caused physicians and public health authorities to take an appraising look at aerobics. If properly implemented and supervised, some of them see it as a possible countermeasure to the Nation's Number One health problem: heart disease.

Heart disease is a national disaster. Every year, nearly a million Americans die from heart and blood vessel disease—a death rate higher than that of any other country. Millions more are crippled by heart attacks. To make matters even worse, the disease appears to be reaching out to younger people. [Men in their 40s and even in their 30s are dropping off at an alarming rate. And, as in everything else, [the women are catching up with the men. Death from heart disease in young American women is also the highest of any country in the world. Perhaps this explains why the longevity of American men ranks 17th and that American women rank tenth among the major nations of the world.

A spokesman for the National Heart Institute sums up the situation in a single sentence: "We're faced with a kind of super-epidemic against which every possible resource must be mobilized."

Exercise, without doubt, is one possible resource.

To claim that aerobics is the only solution to the overwhelming problem of heart disease would be foolish and irresponsible. But I can assure each reader that aerobics— if implemented properly and practiced according to the charts and the rules in this book—will lessen his chance of prematurely developing coronary heart disease or related vascular ailments.

Aside from preventing heart trouble, aerobics holds out other promises for public health. The Russians and Germans have already shown that mass programs of exercise are an efficient way to raise the general fitness level of entire populations.

In the United States, where the vast majority of the population can't pass a basic fitness test, we've got a long way to go in public sponsorship of exercise programs. But the impact of aerobics has nudged a few health officials to look more critically at the role of exercise in preventive medicine.

The state of Vermont, for example, is now using aerobics in a statewide preventive medicine program. And the New York Federal Safety Council recently urged Mayor John V. Lindsay of New York City to set up a municipal aerobics fitness program.

I'm often asked just how many people are practicing aerobics. One way to answer this question would be to refer to book sales—nearly one and one-half million copies of the paperback edition of *Aerobics* have been sold. But book sales cannot be considered an accurate indication of program participation. A better indication comes from the Belden Public Opinion Poll, a regional opinion research organization headquartered in Dallas, Texas. A statewide survey of 60 Texas communities in mid-1968 revealed that 26 percent of the citizens in Texas were exercising regularly and that an estimated 186,000 were following the aerobics program. Projected nationally, this figure indicates that several million Americans may have been practicing aerobics in 1968.

Hundreds of private gyms and health clubs have responded to this mass interest by offering aerobic conditioning courses. The YM-YWCA is leading this trend. In most major cities you can now find at least one branch of the YMCA or YWCA with an aerobics group. So if you seek company, encouragement, advice, and expert supervision for your exercise, the Y is a good place to look.

You might also check the National Jogging Association (P.O. Box 19367, Washington, D.C. 20036), to find out if they have any groups in your vicinity. The Association got off to a fine start in 1968 with a highly suitable ceremony at the Jefferson Memorial in Washington, D.C. Former Secretary of the Interior Stewart L. Udall and Lieutenant General Richard L. Bohannon (ret.), once surgeon general of the USAF, led the assembled crowd in a brisk jog around the reflecting pool.

Another rapidly growing group is called Mile-a-thon International. This organization is supported by the Long Beach Community Hospital, Long Beach, California. They sponsor walking and running activities throughout southern California and once yearly hold a large walking/running event. The emphasis is on participation, not competition, and their appropriate motto is "Witness to Fitness." In 1969, the Mile-a-thon attracted nearly a thousand men, women and children.

Even the interest in cycling seems to be increasing. The League of American Wheelmen, the national amateur cycling organization, reports that bicycle sales in 1968 exceeded all previous years.

But one of the most encouraging recent trends is the growing interest of business and industry in the fitness of their employees. This makes good sense from a management viewpoint. Company-sponsored fitness programs tend to reduce absenteeism, accidents and sick pay. What's more, employees in good physical condition are more alert, more productive, and their morale is higher.

Company fitness programs are rarely restricted to top brass. In most firms, any employee can join. As it turns out, most of them are eager to sign up. A California firm scheduling several aerobics sessions per week polled its employees for their reactions. Here's a typical sampling:

"After a workout, the fog clears," says an airframe designer. "I can focus on what I'm doing."

An accountant comments: "I no longer get drowsy in the afternoon—and I've got plenty of energy left when I get home."

"For me it's like insurance," says an assembly-line inspector. "I just can't afford to get sick. Not with hospital costs a hundred dollars a day."

He has a point. *Staying* well is a lot cheaper than *getting* well.

The general manager of a division of one of the country's largest electronics concerns sums up his experience this way: "Our Division was in serious trouble a while ago due to merger and soft market problems. We now seem to be well on our way towards joining the rest of the corporation in achieving some real success. I give no small credit to your 'Aerobics' program for having provided a management and employee team made up of individuals who feel better, look better, and are more physically and mentally alert."

Such reactions strengthen my hope that the increasing use of aerobics in industry-sponsored programs will become a major factor in building fitness and health throughout the country.

And all of this is just a beginning. The stage has been set for developing aerobics on an even broader scale.

In May 1968, I participated in a seminar at the Congress

of International Military Sports in Fontainebleau, France. At this meeting, plans were laid for aerobics programs within the armed forces of Sweden, Austria, Finland, Korea and Brazil. From the military of these countries, aerobics will surely spread to the civilian population, just as it has in the United States. Moreover, nine countries represented at the congress agreed to pool data obtained in connection with aerobics testing. This will create an international information bank from which valuable new knowledge can be derived.

In little more than a year, aerobics has grown from near obscurity to worldwide scope. It is a deep satisfaction for me to have had a leading part in this development. What greater reward can there be for a research physician than to know that his work has put millions of people on a new road to good health.

2: Revisions and Recaps

DOCTORS LEARN FROM their patients, coaches from their teams, and I've learned a great deal from the thousands of people who have told me about their personal experience with aerobics. Also, I have had the opportunity to collect and evaluate data on many civilian and military personnel including a large United States Air Force aerobics study. At the request of the USAF Chief of Staff, an expanded aerobics project was conducted at five Air Force bases during the period of April–October 1968. A total of 15,146 men were studied, representing one of the largest research projects ever attempted in the field of physical conditioning.

The knowledge gained from this massive research effort and from the public participation in aerobics has helped us formulate new guidelines. No basic principles have been altered. In fact, the original concept of aerobics has been greatly strengthened by the new findings. But we have revised many program details and worked out some new ones. Among them:

- Revised progressive point charts
- Adjustments for different age groups
- New fitness testing rules
- New safety tips
- New sports and exercises added to the aerobic reference charts
- Special pointers for women and children
- Medical examination requirements

DEFINING AEROBICS

Aerobics (pronounced: a-er-ó biks) refers to a variety of exercises that stimulate heart and lung activity for a time period sufficiently long to produce beneficial changes in the body. Running, swimming, cycling, and jogging—these are typical aerobic exercises. There are many others.

15

Aerobics offers you an ample choice of different forms of exercise, including many popular sports. They have one thing in common: by making you work hard, they demand plenty of oxygen. That's the basic idea. That's what makes them aerobic.

The main objective of an aerobic exercise program is to increase the maximum amount of oxygen that the body can process within a given time. This is called your *aerobic capacity*. It is dependent upon an ability to 1) rapidly breathe large amounts of air, 2) forcefully deliver large volumes of blood and 3) effectively deliver oxygen to all parts of the body. In short, it depends upon efficient lungs, a powerful heart, and a good vascular system. Because it reflects the conditions of these vital organs, the aerobic capacity is the best index of overall physical fitness.

TRAINING EFFECT

Collectively, the changes induced by exercise in the various systems and organs of the body are called the *training effect*. Unless the exercise is of sufficient intensity and duration, it will not produce a training effect and cannot be classified as an aerobic exercise. However, this distinction between aerobic and non-aerobic exercises is a laboratory determination, too technical for routine use. Therefore, the point system utilized in the aerobics conditioning program was developed to make this distinction for you. If the program is followed exactly and the required point goals are reached, an adequate training effect is assured. Specifically, aerobic exercise produces a training effect and increases the capacity to utilize oxygen in several ways:

1. It strengthens the muscles of respiration and tends to reduce the resistance to air flow, ultimately facilitating the rapid flow of air in and out of the lungs.
2. It improves the strength and pumping efficiency of the heart, enabling more blood to be pumped with each stroke. This improves the ability to more rapidly transport life-sustaining oxygen from the lungs to the heart and ultimately to all parts of the body.
3. It tones up muscles throughout the body, thereby improving the general circulation, at times lowering blood pressure and reducing the work on the heart.

4. It causes an increase in the total amount of blood circulating through the body and increases the number of red blood cells and the amount of hemoglobin, making the blood a more efficient oxygen carrier.

None of this is speculation. The anatomic and biochemical changes characteristic of the training effect have been documented in the laboratory many times. And throughout this book, reference will be made to many of these studies which have shown the health-building action of the training effect, especially as it concerns the heart.

POINT CHARTS

The training effect is the goal of an aerobic conditioning program. The means for achieving that goal is also provided by the program. That is the purpose of the point charts. Here lies the unique merit of the aerobic system: you can measure your own progress as if you were being monitored in a medical research laboratory. All you need is the point chart and a stopwatch. In effect, aerobics puts the lab in your pocket.

Many people ask, "What is so important about points? Why isn't it sufficient just to add up the total distance you walk or run?"

For an answer, I refer to an experience I had several years ago. Two active runners in their early forties, comparable in weight and height, came to my laboratory for an evaluation on the treadmill. In the interview prior to their evaluation, I discovered that both men were running two miles, five days a week. I immediately assumed that their level of fitness was comparable but was quite surprised at the results of their treadmill test. One of the subjects was clearly in excellent condition and the other barely passed.

Why the difference?

I was perplexed until I asked another question: *"How fast do you run your two miles?"* The first said he averaged between 13:30–14:00 minutes whereas the second took over 20:00 minutes. One was a runner and the other a jogger. It was readily apparent that I needed to consider a factor other than distance—the time.

You achieve a greater training effect if you put more effort into your exercise. Consequently, the point system was developed so that I knew exactly how much effort was being expended.

In hundreds of subsequent studies, we have discovered that it is easy to predict oxygen consumption and fitness based on points but difficult to predict it on miles alone. If you tell me that you are running 20 miles per week, I'm not quite sure what your level of fitness will be, but if you tell me you are averaging 100 points per week, I know that you are in excellent condition!

The aerobic point system was derived from laboratory measurements of the oxygen cost of the exercise, as well as from data obtained in field tests. How these experiments and tests were performed, and how the point charts were calculated, has been explained at length in my earlier book. For the user of these charts all that is necessary is to understand that the aerobic points refer to the energy expended.

The point value assigned to each exercise indicates that amount of oxygen consumed by the body during a particular activity. More points mean more effort expended, that is, more oxygen burned in the body at a faster rate. In short, the point system measures the energy cost of the exercise.

For example, if you run a mile in 11:30 minutes, you can earn 3 points. Run the mile in 8:30 minutes and you earn 4 points.

"Hold it Doc," one of the airmen interrupted when I was explaining this to a test group. "You mean I get more points for exercising less?"

"How so?" I asked, somewhat confused.

"Well, you're giving me 3 points for 11:30 minutes and 4 points for exercising three minutes less, even though the distance is the same."

I finally saw his problem. Throughout the aerobic charts, shorter completion times mean more points. That's what confused him.

"Look at it this way," I explained, "Suppose you're driving your car. To cover a mile faster, you have to step down harder on the gas pedal. Why? Because going faster takes more power from the engine. It's the same when you're running. If you run a mile in a shorter time, your energy output is greater. Your heart and lungs work harder. That's why you get more points for the shorter time span."

Because the point charts let you measure the amount of effort you expend, you can now take exercise in *progressive* doses. And this is vitally important. In fact, it is the key to the aerobic conditioning program. The body must gradually adjust itself to increasing amounts of exercise. Too much too fast can be as damaging as too little too late. That's why the charts for the conditioning program spell out exact exercise rations from week to week. "Why are 30 points per week necessary? Why not 20 or wouldn't 50 be even better?" These are questions that are asked at nearly all of my presentations.

The answer is always the same. From testing and training thousands of men and women, I have been able to show that roughly 80 percent of the people who follow the progressive programs and work up to 30 points per week can reach our minimum standards of fitness.

"And where did you get your standards?"

The standards I have established are based mainly on age-adjusted Swedish standards—and Swedish researchers in exercise physiology have long been recognized as the world's leaders in this field.

AGE CODING

As you may have noticed in the preceding paragraph, I said *age adjusted* standards. And a new feature of this book is not only progressive exercise charts adjusted to age but also new categories of fitness based on age. The breakdown of the four separate age brackets is as follows:

> Under 30
> 30 to 39
> 40 to 49
> 50 and over

Splitting the conditioning programs into four separate training routines permitted me to use a different approach for the older age groups. But the 30 point per week requirement still remains—it just takes a little longer time to reach it.

The original conditioning program was based on data obtained exclusively from my Air Force research group. Their average age was in the middle twenties. After the general public took up aerobics, it became clear that certain modifications were needed. Too many civilians, deskbound, middle aged and maybe a little paunchy, just weren't able to meet exercise norms set up for young airmen.

The physical director of a YMCA branch of mid-Manhattan filed a typical report:

In this location we gets lots of businessmen coming in for exercise. Some of the men in our aerobics group are well into middle age, ranging between 47 and 53. At the outset, they didn't seem in any worse shape than the rest. But they soon found that they couldn't keep up with the younger men or with the chart requirements of the aerobics program. They get discouraged, and some would quit. I hated to see them drop out. After all, they needed the exercise most. Should I have modified the chart requirements for them? If so, how?

Similar letters flowed in by the dozens. In response, I made a special effort to draw older persons into the expanded research program to study their exercise needs. Among them, I even picked several hundred men and women over 50 years of age to evaluate their reactions to the aerobics program. The new age-adjusted charts are the outcome of these studies.

Age is not a major obstacle to fitness. No matter what age bracket you belong to, you can reach a satisfactory level of fitness. But you must work toward the common goal using a different approach and at a different rate.

The new age-coding of the charts, I hope, will open the door to aerobics for even broader segments of the population, particularly those in the over-40 brackets. With aerobics, they can avoid many symptoms of premature aging, regain the vigor and vitality they have long thought lost, and make the "best years of life" just that.

We'll discuss the many new hints and suggestions that have come from our expanding experience with aerobics as we go along. First, let's get started in the new aerobics.

3: The Physical Examination

DIFFERENT PEOPLE HAVE different objectives in their quest for fitness. To an athlete, it's seconds shaved off a mile, or that extra burst of speed in the last minute of the game. To a lawyer, it's alertness after hours of hard bargaining. To a housewife, a dress two sizes smaller, or maybe just the sense of abundant well-being, the positive outlook and re-gained youthfulness that comes from really being "fit."

No matter what your particular exercise aim may be, the most important thing is to achieve it safely. After all, you want to gain your health, not lose it. That's why a thor-ough physical examination should be the very first step on your road to fitness.

Emphasizing the importance of such an examination is the following tragic incident. On July 23, 1968, a leading West Coast newspaper exploded a banner headline: TWO MORE JOGGERS DIE! Other newspapers across the coun-try picked up the story. Occurring shortly after a wave of enthusiasm had made jogging something of a nationwide sport, the tragedy suddenly focused national concern on the problem of safety in exercise.

My phone rang almost constantly. Physicians and lay people alike were anxiously asking under what conditions exercise might be dangerous, and prominent doctors were wondering out loud in newspapers and magazines whether perhaps the idea of exercise had been oversold to the public.

In response to this widespread concern, I decided to investigate more closely the case of the two joggers who had suffered fatal heart attacks during the exercise. Both, it turnd out, had severe heart disease, and one of them had been told by a prominent West Coast physician that he should under no circumstances engage in vigorous exercise. Yet, contrary to medical advice, the man started jogging at a strenuous rate, mistakenly believing that this would help him overcome his heart condition more quickly. In-

21

stead, jogging at a hard pace strained his weak heart beyond its limits.

The one good thing growing out of this tragedy was the realization on the part of physicians that anyone enter-ing an exercise or physical conditioning program should have a medical checkup before starting. So before you embark on any exercise program, get your doctor's approval.

MEDICAL CHECKUP

Because no standards have yet been set for this pre-exercise checkup, many doctors have asked for recommended procedures. In response to these inquiries, I collaborated with several of my colleagues and wtih the AMA Committee on Physical Fitness and Exercise to define the kind of ex-amination recommended for this purpose. The full medical details are to be published in a scientific article entitled "Guidelines in the Management of the Exercising Patient." The main objective of this examination is to spot heart, lung, and blood vessel problems that could make exercise potentially dangerous. This is especially important for older persons who are more likely to be affected by such prob-lems.

The following guidelines are proposed for different age groups:

Under 30: You can start exercising if you've had a check-up within the past year and the doctor found nothing wrong with you.

Between 30 and 39: You should have a checkup within three months before you start exercising. The examination should include an electrocardiogram (ECG) taken at rest.

Between 40 and 59: Same as for the 30–39 group with one important addition. Your doctor should also take an ECG to check your heart while you are exercising. Your pulse rate during this test should approach the level it would during aerobic workouts.*

Over 59: The same requirements as for the 40–59 age group except that the examination should be performed immediately before embarking on any exercise program.

* For detailed requirements, physicians may refer to the Appendix for a chart listing the target heart rates to be used in taking an exercise ECG.

The trouble is that not many doctors are equipped to take ECGs during exercise. Ideally, they should have either a stationary bicycle or a treadmill in their office so that they can continuously monitor your ECG while you vigorously exercise. With growing popular interest in exercise, I hope that more doctors will install this kind of equipment. After all, a good stationary bicycle with adjustable brake force costs less than $100. A treadmill is more expensive.

If your doctor doesn't have this kind of equipment, he can still take your ECG while you are under stress by giving you a variant of the so-called Masters two-step test. In this test you rapidly go up and down a single step until your pulse rate reaches the required level. The ECG and pulse should be monitored both during and after such exercise. Occasionally ECG changes produced by the exercise stress do not show up until two to five minutes after the exercise has stopped. That's why the ECG should continue to be monitored during the recovery period.

The purpose of these tests is to spot any heart condition that might cause trouble during exercise. If coronary weakness or some other defect shows up, exercise must be scaled down to levels of physical demand that your heart can meet safely. Your doctor may suggest that you do your exercising in a special medically supervised program until you have made sufficient improvement to continue on your own. In fact, he may recommend that you confine yourself to walking—no running, jogging or other more strenuous forms of exercise.

Don't feel discouraged about this. Done consistently and according to the aerobic charts, walking can gain for you the same benefits as any of the more strenuous exercises. The only difference is that it takes a little longer. Even if you do nothing but walk, you can eventually be as aerobically fit as anyone.

While walking can be recommended to almost anyone, the more vigorous exercises, notably jogging and running, are strictly prohibited for persons suffering from any of the following conditions:

1. Moderate to severe coronary heart disease causing chest pain with minimal activity (angina pectoris).

2. Recent heart attacks. You must wait at least three months after a heart attack before starting on a regular exercise program. Even then your exercise program must be medically supervised.

3. Severe disease of the heart valves, primarily as a result of old rheumatic fever. Some patients of this type should not exercise at all—not even to the extent of fast walking.

4. Certain types of congenital heart disease, particularly those in which the surface of the body turns blue during exercise.

5. Greatly enlarged heart due to high blood pressure or other types of progressive heart disease.

6. Severe irregularities of the heartbeat requiring medication or frequent medical attention.

7. Uncontrolled sugar diabetes constantly fluctuating from too much to not enough blood sugar.

8. High blood pressure not controlled by medication; *i.e.,* blood pressure exceeding 180/110 even with medication.

9. Excessive obesity. If you are more than 35 pounds overweight according to the standard weight charts, you must lose weight on a walking program before you can begin running or jogging.

10. Any infectious disease during its acute stage.

Another group of ailments do not prevent you from exercising altogether but make it necessary to proceed with caution and under medical supervision. In contrast to the above-named conditions, which are absolute *contraindications,* the following are regarded—medically speaking—as *relative* contraindications:

1. Any infectious disease in its convalescent or chronic stage.

2. Sugar diabetes controlled by insulin.

3. A history of recent or active internal bleeding. (Some of these patients should not exercise at all.)

4. Kidney disease, either chronic or acute.

5. Anemia under treatment but not yet corrected (less than 10 grams of hemoglobin).

6. Acute or chronic lung disease resulting in breathing difficulty with even light exercise.

7. Elevated blood pressure which can be lowered only to 150/90 with medication.
8. Blood vessel disease of the legs that produces pain with walking.
9. Arthritis in the back, legs, feet or ankles, requiring frequent medication for relief of pain.
10. Convulsive disease not completely controlled with medication.

Let me stress once more that these relative contraindications do not rule out exercise. To the contrary, in some cases exercise helps reduce their symptoms. But medical judgment and supervision must be applied to each individual case.

AGE RESTRICTIONS

As you grow in years, the efficiency of your heart and lungs gradually decreases. One of the benefits of aerobic exercise is that it slows down this aspect of aging and to some degree helps you retain your youthful fitness. But if you have not been exercising regularly, you should observe certain age restrictions when you consider starting a conditioning program.

Up to 30 years of age: Unless you have some obvious medical problem, you can enter any type of an exercise program—running, jogging, swimming, cycling—no restrictions. Just choose one that you enjoy.

Between 30 and 50 years of age: You're still good for almost everything. You have your choice of sports. But if you plan to do some of the more strenuous exercises, be sure to get your doctor's specific approval of your decision.

Between 50 and 59 years: It would be better if you started a walking program. Only after you have conditioned yourself by walking according to the charts should you consider running, jogging, or more demanding competitive sports such as basketball, handball, or squash. Have your doctor check you out again before you start such activities. Othrwise you're better off sticking with less arduous exercises, such as walking, golf, cycling (particularly stationary cycling), and swimming.

Age 60 and over: If you're like most people in this age group, avoid jogging, running and vigorous competitive sports. Walking, swimming and stationary cycling will do you a lot more good.

However, there are exceptions for the over-60 bracket. If you have been keeping in shape by regular exercise for many years so that you have built up and maintained your aerobic capacity, you may safely participate in such vigorous activities as jogging, running, and stationary running. You're also free to engage in more strenuous activities if you do your exercise in a medically supervised group.

If you doubt that regular conditioning exercise can keep you fit way beyond 60, look at 102-year-old Larry Lewis. He's been exercising practically all his life, first as a member of Ringling Brothers and Barnum and Bailey's circus, and since the age of 80, as a regular jogger. Now he is on his feet some eight hours each day as a banquet waiter at San Francisco's St. Francis Hotel.

Larry runs six miles every morning in Golden Gate Park. Then he walks five miles to work, and after his long shift, he usually walks home. On his 102nd birthday he added something extra to this routine. He ran a 100-yard dash in 17.3 seconds—0.5 faster than he was able to do it at the age of 101. It's not official, but I'm pretty sure that this is the world record for the 100-yard dash for men above one hundred years of age!

In this chapter, I have stressed the need for a medical examination prior to entering *any* exercise program, because as a physician it is my duty to warn against possible health risks. But the encouraging fact is that the great majority of people pass their pre-exercise examination with no trouble at all and can enter sensible exercise programs without reservation.

Because of incidents like the death of the California joggers, people sometimes get the idea that all exercise is risky. They think exercise killed those joggers. Exactly the opposite is true. They died because of the severity of their disease whereas proper exercise might have strengthened their hearts and saved their lives—if they had followed reasonable medical advice.

Exercise is the medicine that keeps countless people alive. But like all medicine, it must be taken according to prescription.

4: Fitness Testing and Categories

FITNESS TESTING IS strictly optional. You can put yourself in fine shape without ever taking any test at all. Just follow the conditioning charts. By the time you reach the 30-points-per-week level, just take it for granted that you're in good condition.

Yet, there are many occasions when physical fitness testing is extremely useful. For example, physicians may need to know a patient's level of fitness so that they can determine the amount of physical activity he may safely perform on the job. Coaches may want to test the fitness of individual athletes or even their entire team before starting into seasonal competition. Physical educators may benefit from evaluating their classes as a means of determining their response to a particular training program. Even if you are exercising strictly on your own, you may want to find out just where you stand in comparison with others. Or once you start an exercise program, you may want a method for monitoring your progress.

For all these purposes, we have developed aerobic fitness tests that are both simple and accurate. Basically, the tests measure your aerobic capacity—the maximum amount of oxygen your body can process during exhausting work. This is one of the best, if not the best available indicator of general fitness and physical capability.

MEASURING AEROBIC CAPACITY

The groundwork for developing an aerobic fitness test was done in the laboratory. To measure a man's aerobic capacity, we ask him to walk/run on a motor driven treadmill. Its speed can be varied from a slow walk to a quick dash, and the incline can be raised to simulate an uphill run. The man on the treadmill has no choice but to move at the speed set by the technician. If he doesn't run hard enough, he falls off backwards. That's how we were able to encourage our volunteers to run up to the point of exhaustion—assuring a maximum effort.

During these tests we continuously monitored the electrocardiogram and blood pressure to guard against overexertion. At the first sign of excessive heart strain, we stopped the test. By watching the electrocardiogram, blood pressure and respiration rate, we could also tell whether our test subject was really working to the limit of his capacity.

While the test subjects were running on the treadmill, they breathed into a one-way valve that enabled us to collect the air they exhaled. This air was then analyzed to determine the amount of oxygen their bodies utilized during their exhausting effort. This amount (measured in milliliters per kilogram of total body weight per minute) marks a man's aerobic capacity. It is his fitness index.

Through these lab tests we found, for example, that a man less than 29 years of age and in good physical condition can process upward of 42.5 milliliters of oxygen per kilogram per minute, while a person in very poor shape can process only 25 milliliters or less.

On the basis of these measurements we set up the following five Fitness Categories for men:

Fitness Category	Oxygen Consumption (Ml/Kg/Min)			
	Under 30	*30–39*	*40–49*	*50+*
I. Very Poor	< 25.0	< 25.0	< 25.0	
II. Poor	25.0–33.7	25.0–30.1	25.0–26.4	< 25.0
III. Fair	33.8–42.5	30.2–39.1	26.5–35.4	25.0–33.7
IV. Good	42.6–51.5	39.2–48.0	35.5–45.0	33.8–43.0
V. Excellent	51.6+	48.1+	45.1+	43.1+

< Means less than.

FIELD TESTING

So much for theory. Obviously, this type of laboratory fitness testing is necessary for research but it isn't very practical. It takes about $10,000 worth of equipment, three technicians and an hour's time to test a single person. For general use, simpler field testing methods had to be developed. Fortunately, we were able to devise field tests requiring only a stop watch and a place to run. Despite their simplicity and ease of administration these field tests are almost as accurate and reliable as laboratory measurements made on the treadmill.

Since your heart rate and blood pressure cannot be monitored continuously during a field test, there is a certain risk if you take such a test without having been properly conditioned by previous exercise. That is why I suggest the following precautions:

1. Don't take a fitness test prior to beginning an exercise program if you are over 30 years of age.

2. Be sure to have a medical examination, as outlined in Chapter 3, before you take a fitness test. If you are over 30, it is still safer to postpone the test until you have completed the six-week "starter program" as described in Chapter Six.

3. If you comply with the above, yet experience extreme fatigue, shortness of breath, light-headedness or nausea during the physical fitness test, stop immediately. Do not try to repeat the test until your fitness level has been gradually improved through regular exercise.

12-MINUTE TEST

The first of these field tests is the 12-minute test. Run and walk as far as you comfortably can in 12 minutes. If you get winded, slow down awhile until you get your breath back. Then run again for a stretch. The idea is to cover the greatest distance you can in those 12 minutes. Our findings show that the distance covered correlates very accurately (coefficient of correlation = .90) with treadmill measurements of oxygen consumption and aerobic capacity. In other words, you can measure your aerobic capacity and determine your fitness category simply by a 12-minute run.

The correlation between distance covered in 12 minutes and oxygen consumption works out as follows:

DISTANCE COVERED (Miles)	OXYGEN CONSUMPTION (Ml/Kg/Min)
less than 1.0	less than 25.0
1.0 to 1.24	25.0 to 33.7
1.25 to 1.49	33.8 to 42.5
1.50 to 1.74	42.6 to 51.5
1.75 miles or more	51.6 or more

(Data based on men 17–52 years of age)

If you have no other way to measure how far you have run, you can do it by driving the same stretch of road in your car and reading the distance covered on the odometer. Don't try to measure distance with a pedometer. We've checked out several and none are sufficiently accurate.

The following charts tell you how to rate yourself on the 12-minute test, and in contrast to previously published test charts, these have been adjusted for different age groups. The original 12-minute test chart was designed for male Air Force personnel whose average age was under 30. But since so many people past 30 have expressed interest in the aerobics program, it has become necessary to establish some age-adjusted standards for both men and women. These new factors have been incorporated in the revised charts. As they stand now, these charts are applicable to a broad spectrum of the population, although the chart for women is a preliminary chart only.

12-Minute Test for Men

(Distances in miles covered in 12-minutes)

Fitness Category	Age			
	Under 30	*30–39*	*40–49*	*50+*
I. Very Poor	< 1.0	< .95	< .85	< .80
II. Poor	1.0–1.24	.95–1.14	.85–1.04	.80– .99
III. Fair	1.25–1.49	1.15–1.39	1.05–1.29	1.0 –1.24
IV. Good	1.50–1.74	1.40–1.64	1.30–1.54	1.25–1.49
V. Excellent	1.75+	1.65+	1.55+	1.50+

< Means less than.

12-Minute Test for Women *

(Distance in miles covered in 12 minutes)

Fitness Category	Age			
	Under 30	*30–39*	*40–49*	*50+*
I. Very Poor	< .95	< .85	< .75	< .65
II. Poor	.95–1.14	.85–1.04	.75– .94	.65– .84
III. Fair	1.15–1.34	1.05–1.24	.95–1.14	.85–1.04
IV. Good	1.35–1.64	1.25–1.54	1.15–1.44	1.05–1.34
V. Excellent	1.65+	1.55+	1.45+	1.35+

* Preliminary chart based on limited data.
< Means less than.

1.5 MILE TEST

During the summer of 1968, I was asked to evaluate the physical fitness of more than 15,000 members of the Air Force. For testing such a large group, the 12-minute test described above proved too cumbersome. It was impossible to monitor a thousand men on a single track in a morning, as was required by our tight schedule. Some modification of test procedures had to be made.

To simplify the administration of the test to large groups, we took the information we had accumulated from the 12-minute test and developed new standards based on the time required to run 1.5 miles. The five fitness categories were then related to the age of the subject as well as the time required to run the 1.5 mile distance. If you prefer this type of test to the 12-minute test, rate yourself according to the following charts:

1.5 MILE TEST FOR MEN †

(Running time in minutes for 1.5 mile distance)

FITNESS CATEGORY	AGE			
	Under 30	30–39	40–49	50+
I. Very Poor	16:30+	17:30+	18:30+	19:00+
II. Poor	16:30— 14:31	17:30— 15:31	18:30— 16:31	19:00— 17:01
III. Fair	14:30— 12:01	15:30— 13:01	16:30— 14:01	17:00— 14:31
IV. Good	12:00— 10:16	13:00— 11:01	14:00— 11:31	14:30— 12:01
V. Excellent *	<10:15	<11:00	<11:30	<12:00

† No separate chart is provided for women because available data are still too tentative.

* For military personnel, the Excellent requirements are 15–30 seconds faster.

< Means less than.

With the aid of these field tests we have been able to confirm the effects of aerobic training in thousands of Air Force personnel. Typically, a deconditioned man in the Very Poor category with an aerobic capacity of less than 25 milliliters can increase his capacity by as much as 30 percent in response to aerobic conditioning.

I strongly urge coaches and sports instructors to employ either the 12-minute or the 1.5-mile tests in place of some of the older methods. Many athletic teams will test their athletes by asking them to run one mile or the even shorter distance of 600 yards. Usually the requirement is to run the mile in less than six or seven minutes. If an athlete can do this, he supposedly has sufficient endurance capacity.

The irony is that the one-mile run—let alone the 600-yard run—is much too short to accurately test for endurance or aerobic capacity. Such relatively brief spurts are basically tests of anaerobic capacity; *i.e.* the ability to perform at a high level of energy output for very short periods. It is a poor indicator of the athlete's ability to finish the game without slackening off toward the end. Our observation that a one-mile run does not represent a significant challenge to an athlete's aerobic capacity has recently been confirmed by other researchers. A run of at least 1.5 miles or a duration of at least 12 minutes is necessary to estimate accurately by field-testing methods the maximum oxygen consumption.

An increasing number of athletic teams have been using both the 12-minute and the 1.5-mile tests in conjunction with their off-season and in-season conditioning. The University of Nebraska football team, for example, found that less than half of their men were able to run 1.5 miles in under 12:00 minutes at the beginning of spring training. Yet at the end of spring training, they proudly announced that every man on the team—including the heavy tackles—was able to run 1.5 miles in 12 minutes or less.

Calvert Hall High School, Towson, Maryland, employed intensive aerobic conditioning prior to the football season, then used the 12-minute test weekly during the season to assure that team members were keeping up their fitness. For the first time in the history of the school, the team went through the entire season without time lost due to injuries, indicating that the fitness and added alertness gained from aerobics may be an important factor in avoiding athletic injury. The Green Bay Packers professional football team have publicized the fact that they use aerobics during the off-season. They hope that this off-season conditioning will improve their performance in season by: 1) increasing the stamina and endurance of their players; 2) reducing athletic injuries; and 3) increasing the number of years a player can actively participate as a team member.

FITNESS COMPARISONS

The 12-minute and 1.5-mile tests now, for the first time, provide a practical method for measuring and comparing the fitness of large numbers of people. As these tests become more widely used, we may expect interesting new information about fitness levels at different schools, in different occupations, different states and countries. Such data will be valuable in developing aerobic exercise programs aimed at raising the general level of fitness for men and women of all ages.

One of the first foreign surveys of this kind was made by Arthur Zechner, a captain in the Austrian army. He gave the 12-minute test to 1157 recruits whose average age was 19 years. Here are the results:

1157 AUSTRIAN MALES—INITIAL TESTING

(18–20 Years of Age)

FITNESS CATEGORY	Percent
I. Very Poor	0.6
II. Poor	3.6
III. Fair	20.5
IV. Good	44.5
V. Excellent	30.8

Contrast these findings with our own Air Force personnel in the same age group:

1370 AMERICAN MALES—INITIAL TESTING

(18–20 Years of Age)

FITNESS CATEGORY	Percent
I. Very Poor	3.0
II. Poor	6.7
III. Fair	31.2
IV. Good	52.8
V. Excellent	6.3

The figures speak pretty well for themselves. In Austria, walking and cycling are still common means of transportation, and country hikes are a favorite Sunday activity. We may have better transportation and fancier entertainment, but they don't make us any healthier.

Captain Zechner also used the 12-minute fitness test to compare the performance of smokers and nonsmokers in this group of young men. He found that men smoking as few as *five* cigarettes a day showed an impairment in their running performance, added proof that smoking and fitness don't mix.

FIELD TESTING EXPERIENCE

The field tests described in this chapter have been studied by a number of investigators over the past two years and have been found substantially safe and efficient.

In terms of sheer numbers, my own experience in fitness testing probably exceeds that of any other researcher. In the course of developing the USAF Aerobics Physical Fitness Program, I supervised 12-minute and 1.5-mile tests on more than 30,000 men and women, both in the laboratory and in the field. Only a single serious incident occurred during this whole testing effort. A 51-year-old man suffered a heart attack 30 minutes following a 1.5-mile test.

I can't say with absolute assurance that this heart attack would not have occurred if proper safeguards had been observed. However if, prior to the initial test, this man had been given a medical examination as outlined in Chapter Three, some sign of heart disease might have been evident. He would then have been advised not to participate in any fitness test.

If the precautions set forth in this book are followed, fitness testing carries virtually no risk and is a valuable part of a physical training program. By monitoring the progress of athletic teams or other groups engaged in physical conditioning, it provides an excellent guide for coach and player alike.

However, let me repeat that a person exercising on his own and interested only in improving his personal fitness need not take any fitness test at all. If he just keeps on earning the number of aerobic points set forth in the conditioning charts, he'll achieve a good level of fitness with or without testing.

5: Entering the Aerobics Program

Two WEEKS AGO my phone rang. A long distance call from Nebraska.

"Dr. Cooper?"

"Speaking."

"Well, I have a complaint about aerobics," a rather disgruntled voice said at the other end. "I've been on the program six weeks and now my legs are so sore I can hardly move."

"What program did you start?" I asked.

"Running."

"Did you walk for a couple of weeks before you started running?"

"Oh no. I started running the first day and by the end of the first week I ran a mile in nine minutes."

That's when I had my first inkling of what was wrong with the fellow. To confirm my theory, I asked: "How fast were you going after three weeks?"

"I ran a mile in seven minutes," he said proudly. "And by the time my legs gave out after six weeks, I got it down to six minutes and thirty seconds."

No wonder he was in trouble. He ignored the first rule of aerobics: never get ahead of yourself—or of the charts!

PROGRESS SLOWLY

Most of us are always trying to get there in a hurry—wherever we may be going. In exercise this just doesn't work and merely invites trouble. Don't rush your conditioning program. Work up to your goal gradually.

I discourage people from starting directly on a running program unless they have been exercising regularly. All three of the progressive running programs require at least one week of walking before any running. Working up slowly to more strenuous effort is important not only to accustom the heart to the new demands but also to let tendons and muscles adjust themselves to the new activity.

WARM UP PROPERLY

Any athlete knows that the body doesn't spring suddenly into high gear from a state of rest. It needs a period of gradual warm-up before strenuous effort, in order to minimize muscle and joint problems. This is particularly important for people past 40.

I usually recommend the following five-minute routine: During the first minute do stretching exercises for arms, legs and back. During the second minute do sit-ups (with your knees bent) and push-ups. During the third minute, walk in a circle at a fairly rapid pace. During the fourth minute alternate 15 seconds of walking with 15 seconds of jogging— a sort of half-run. During the fifth minute jog continuously; *i.e.* run at a very slow speed—approximately at the rate of a 12- 13-minute mile.

Stay flat-footed as much as possible during your warm-up run. That will give the tendons in your feet and ankles a chance to stretch gradually, helping to avoid possible irritation from sudden stress.

After this five-minute routine, start your regular aerobic workout. If you are about to participate in some kind of endurance activity, *e.g.*, a three-mile run, the running part of the warm-up may be incorporated into the first few minutes of the activity itself.

EXERCISE WITHIN YOUR TOLERANCE

One basic rule to be aware of in entering an exercise program is this: Avoid straining and pushing yourself to the extent that you become overly fatigued. Such intense effort at the outset of an exercise program is not only dangerous, it also defeats your basic purpose. Instead of feeling more fit and more vigorous, you'll just feel chronically tired.

COOL DOWN SLOWLY

While a warm-up is a generally accepted practice, few people realize that the body also needs a cooling-down period after exercise. They slump into complete relaxation immediately after exercise. This can cause dizzy spells, fainting and even more serious consequences. Strange as it seems you must get ready for rest.

Five minutes of walking or very slow jogging eases the transition between running and resting.

One dramatic experiment performed back in 1941 documented the importance of cooling down after a workout. One hundred men were asked to run to exhaustion on a treadmill. Then they were told to stand motionless. Seventeen of them promptly fainted. What caused this effect?

Immediately after running, most of the blood was pooled in their legs. Without a gradual cool-down period they couldn't get enough blood back to where it was needed— the heart and the brain. The blood stayed in their legs and they blacked out.

A similar incident occurred to an acquaintance of mine. He was on a vacation trip to Washington, D.C., and being an ardent aerobics fan, he spurned the elevators in the Washington monument and climbed all the way to the top. Then he walked all the way down. Nothing happened.

The next day he climbed the more than 900 steps to the top again—just to keep himself in shape. As he reached the top, it just so happened that the elevator door opened for a ride back down. His willpower sagged momentarily, and he accepted the mute invitation of the open elevator door for the down-trip. As soon as the elevator reached the ground floor, he fainted.

Rushed to the hospital by anxious bystanders, he soon recovered but was kept there for observation for several days. The doctors ran all sorts of tests on him, suspecting heart irregularities and other ailments. But none of the tests showed anything abnormal. Finally, perplexed, he contacted me by phone. After hearing the details of his fainting episode, I immediately suspected what had happened. He very likely collapsed because of an insufficient cool-down period. Standing motionless in the crowded elevator, he suffered the same symptoms as the men whose vigorous treadmill exercise was followed by a sudden standstill. Fortunately, the episode produced no lasting damage and he was able to continue his aerobic program without problems.

Another man was less lucky. He was a well-conditioned,

47-year-old man who had been running regularly for three months. Usually he would trot at a slow pace for 3–5 minutes after his run, allowing his body to relax gradually. But one day because of very cold weather, he sat down in his warm car immediately after the run. He was found slumped over the steering wheel.

What happened is a matter of speculation, since the autopsy did not reveal the cause of his death. However, sudden relaxation, plus the warmth of his car may have combined lethally. The blood had shifted to the legs during the run. At the sudden stop of activity, the muscles no longer helped return the blood to the heart. To make matters worse, the capillary vessels were dilated by the sudden warmth in the car. The heart and brain were suddenly without adequate blood supply, causing heart stoppage. This tragic incident again underlines the importance of two basic precautions:

1. Taper off gradually. Trot or walk for a few minutes after any strenuous exercise, preferably at the same air temperature as that at which the exercise was performed.

2. Avoid going into a hot room or a hot shower immediately after exercise. Wait until you cool down and have stopped sweating before you shower. About the worst thing you can do is to go into a steamroom or sauna immediately after a hard, hot workout.

CALISTHENICS

Because I favor aerobic exercise as the basic requirement for fitness, some readers of my earlier book concluded that I advise against calisthenics. This is definitely not so. It's not an either/or proposition. If you do aerobics, that doesn't rule out calisthenics. Both are good, but each serves a different purpose. Calisthenics builds agility, coordination and muscular strength, particularly in the arms and the upper torso. Aerobics builds basic fitness and endurance. A highly conditioned person needs both.

I do a certain amount of calisthenics in addition to aerobics: sit-ups with the knees bent, toe-touches and push-ups. I recommend doing such calisthenics either before or after aerobic workouts, particularly if the aerobic exercise involves mainly the legs and does not directly engage the muscles of the upper body. The warm-up or cool-down periods are convenient periods for doing such calisthenics.

WHEN TO EXERCISE

You can bolster your willpower by always exercising at the same time of day. Some people like getting their aerobics out of the way first thing in the morning.

Others claim that they can't exercise in the morning because "my body is slow to awaken." I can find no medical evidence in support of this. But for whatever reasons, some people feel sluggish in the morning. They are the so-called "evening types" who don't really come alive until later in the day. Many of them prefer exercise in the late afternoon or evening.

Still others use their lunch hour as an exercise period.

Lunch-hour exercise has a special advantage for weight watchers. Vigorous activity tends to suppress appetite immediately afterward. Therefore, lunch hour athletes may find that they can get by without lunch—"just a bowl of soup or a cold drink." The combined effect of exercise and reduced food intake soon gets rid of those extra pounds and inches.

"Exercise cuts down appetite?" people ask in surprise. "I thought it would make you hungry!"

True, moderate exercise may increase the appetite. But intense exercise for even relatively short periods—such as most aerobic workouts—decreases appetite. Such exercise shunts the blood away from your stomach. As a result, you don't have much of a desire for food. Even after you've recovered from the exercise, your appetite rarely increases above normal. The net result is that you tend to eat less without feeling hungry.

A sergeant at Lackland Air Force Base was about 40 pounds overweight. He had never been able to follow a diet. In addition to eating big meals, he was always snacking between meals. I suggested aerobic workouts just before lunch. The results were excellent. In five weeks, he lost 20 pounds by merely skipping lunch and exercising.

Late afternoon exercise also has certain advantages. Because it dispels tension, after-office exercise is especially helpful to men whose jobs put them under nervous strain. It works as a very effective tranquilizer. People with ulcers and other nervous disturbances often find that after-work exercise greatly reduces their symptoms.

Several people have asked about exercising vigorously after dinner. They like to wait until the day cools. I tell them that it doesn't really matter when you exercise, as long as you wait at least two hours after a meal.

I know people who exercise just before bedtime. Afterwards they feel relaxed and pleasantly tired and drop right off to sleep. That's fine if you can do it. For most people it doesn't work out that way. Exercise gets them physically too agitated to be able to sleep immediately afterward. They need a quiet unwinding period of one to two hours between exercise and sleep.

One thing about exercising late in the day: for some reason it seems to encourage quitting. Bill Bowerman, track coach at the University of Oregon, kept a record on dropouts in a large group of joggers over a period of several years. The quitting rate among morning joggers was less than 30 percent. Among the afternoon and evening joggers it was more than 60 percent.

Why is quitting more prevalent among the afternoon and evening men? I have no medical explanation, but I have a hunch that it is easier to find an excuse for not exercising in the afternoon than it is at 6:00 A.M.

When I discussed early-morning exercise at the International Congress on Military Sports at Fontainebleau, France, some French doctors immediately raised a question: "Exercise before breakfast?" Eating comes first, they insisted.

They have a point. A little sustenance might be preferable, providing it is followed by a sufficient waiting period before the start of exercise. But for most people that is impractical. They haven't got that much time in the morning.

My own experience shows that exercise on an empty stomach does no harm. In our Air Force test group we had thousands of people exercising daily before breakfast without any ill effect. But if you feel that you need to have something in the morning to give you a little quick energy before your workout, I suggest the following: Drink a glass of orange juice; wait 10–15 minutes; then go. To sum up the question of when to exercise, I'd like to make this suggestion: Pick any time that suits your schedule and your needs. The important thing is to make it a regular routine. We are creatures of habit. So let the force of habit help you maintain your exercise pattern.

REGULARITY

If you can't exercise regularly, you're better off not exercising at all. That may sound harsh. But regularity in exercise is an important safety precaution. Now-and-then exercise will not help you build and keep your fitness. It will not increase your aerobic capacity. It will not strengthen your heart so that it can stand a really tough workout.

A case in point was a young Air Force major who liked to play handball whenever he had a chance. Unfortunately, he was able to play only once a week or less. In-between he had no exercise whatsoever.

In the middle of a fast game, he experienced severe chest pain, apparently the result of insufficient blood to the heart. He was taken to the hospital where he spent several weeks although a definite diagnosis was never made.

After his discharge from the hospital, I didn't tell him to quit handball, which he obviously enjoyed, but I advised him to build up his aerobic capacity by doing other exercises between his weekly handball games.

He started cycling and swimming every other day. In response to these closely spaced regular workouts, his aerobic capacity increased to the level where he can now safely and comfortably keep his weekly handball date. While regularity of exercise is important, you should interrupt your exercise program whenever you become ill or excessively fatigued. Avoid vigorous exercise for a 24-hour period after an immunization.

CATCHING UP

But suppose you have to go off on a business trip. Or you come down with a cold. What about these unavoidable interruptions of your exercise routine? How do you catch up?

A lot of people try to pick up where they left off. But that usually proves too strenuous. Your aerobic capacity backslides during a period of inactivity—especially if you're in the upper age brackets.

When you resume exercising after an interruption, you'll have to backtrack on the charts. The question is, how far.

Because different individuals lose aerobic capacity at a different rate during periods of inactivity, you'll have to gauge this for yourself. The main point is, don't push yourself too hard to get back to where you were before.

Wanting to make up for lost time, you might be tempted to overstrain yourself. Fortunately, there are three simple ways to tell if you are exercising too hard during any stage of your conditioning program.

Check 1: Symptoms during exercise

Signs of overexertion during exercise are: tightness or pain in the chest, severe breathlessness, lightheadedness, dizziness, loss of muscle control and nausea. When you experience any of these symptoms, stop exercising immediately.

Check 2: Recovery heart rate

Five minutes after exercise, count your pulse. If it's still over 120, it's a sign that the exercise was too tough for a person in your condition. Ten minutes after exercise, check your pulse again. It should be back below 100. If it isn't let up a little on your exercise program.

The best way to take your pulse is to feel it at your throat. Most people can't feel their own wrist pulse strongly enough for an accurate count. Use a watch with a sweep second hand. Count the pulse for ten seconds, then multiply by six. Or count for 15 seconds and multiply by four.

Check 3: Recovery breathing rate

If you find yourself still short of breath ten minutes after you stop exercising, you can pretty well take it for granted that you're trying too hard. (Normal, resting, respiratory rates range from 12–16 breaths per minute.)

Use these safety checks whenever you think that you might be overexerting.

TEMPERATURE RESTRICTIONS

During extremely hot or extremely cold weather, do not exercise to the point of exhaustion, particularly if you are just starting your conditioning program. The ideal exercise weather is 40° F to 85° F with the humidity less than 60 percent and the wind velocity less than 15 mph. Above or below these limits, reduce the duration and intensity of your exercise.

"But what if the thermometer climbs above 85° F? Should I stop exercising completely?" The answer is a qualified "No!" To some extent you can counteract the effects of heat.

Schedule your exercise in the cooler hours of the morning or evening, at least until you are acclimated.

If you sweat profusely (and this is a characteristic of conditioning), you must increase your salt intake. You can do this either by taking one or two salt tablets with your meals or simply increasing the amount of salt you put on your food. Drink lots of water after working out in a hot and humid environment. That's just as important as getting enough salt. Orange juice and liquid salt solutions are also good fluids to use when sweating excessively.

If there's a sudden heat wave, or if you move to a hotter climate, slow down for at least two weeks to give your body a chance to acclimate itself.

But once the thermometer tops 95 degrees, the best possible advice is to stop all strenuous aerobic exercise. Under conditions of high humidity (above 80 percent), stop when the temperature exceeds 90. Hot and humid weather puts an extra strain on the heart.

Wear light, loose clothing. To avoid chafing, use vaseline or other types of lubricants on the skin areas likely to be affected—particularly the insides of the thighs.

About the worst possible thing you can do is to wear rubberized or other impervious clothing while exercising in hot weather. Rubber suits are advertised as aids to weight reduction. The idea is to work up a sweat in these airtight suits which will enable you to take off weight rapidly. Of course, you gain all those liquid pounds right back as soon as you quench your thirst.

I know of one case involving a heavily overweight businessman in his forties who ran himself nearly to exhaustion in a rubber suit on a hot day, hoping to sweat off a chunk of his midriff. At the end of his run, he collapsed. On his arrival at the hospital he had a temperature above 108° F and only by immediate and competent medical attention was it possible to save his life. Such damaging effects may be due to heat alone but are frequently the result of heat and humidity. Lately, attempts have been made to express both these factors by a single measure, such as the T.H.I. (Temperature-Humidity Index) used by the weather bureau or the H.S.I. (Heat-Stress Index). There is a section in the appendix showing how to determine the severity of the heat stress (WBGT) and a chart detailing exercise limitations advisable when the WBGT reaches certain points.

Cold weather is less dangerous, though by no means harmless. Curiously, people seem more concerned about cold weather than about hot.

Joggers, particularly, can't stand the idea of sitting out the winter. "A day without jogging," one of them writes, "is incomplete to me. I just don't feel right without it. Will jogging in the cold air frostbite my lungs?" he asks.

If anything "frostbites," it will be his ears or his nose, not his lungs. By the time the air gets down into the chest, it's adequately warmed, even if you breathe mainly through your mouth when you exercise.

If the temperature drops below zero, the normal air-warming mechanism of your body may no longer be sufficient, especially if you're heading into an icy wind. Under those conditions too much cold air may be rushing down your windpipe to be adequately warmed. It won't frostbite your lungs, but it may cause constriction of the coronary arteries. (The exact action of the cold air on the circulatory system is not yet fully understood. Research in this area is still under way at the National Heart Institute.)

That's probably what happens to people who suffer heart attacks while shoveling snow in icy air. Of course, most of them are in poor condition to begin with. They exhaust themselves by shoveling, and the added strain imposed by the cold air is more than they can tolerate.

Some of our Air Force personnel in Alaska ran throughout the winter without difficulty, showing that cold weather is no deterrent to exercise if one is physically fit, and if sensible safeguards are taken. One of these is cooling down very gradually after you've worked up a sweat. Don't allow yourself to get chilled. Another is putting a scarf over your mouth to help warm up the air. Of course, the fabric has to be loose-knit for fairly free air passage. A dental or surgical mask also works well for this purpose. And always let someone know when and where you will be exercising.

Summing up cold weather precautions, I'm not saying that you should quit outdoor exercise when the weather gets below freezing, but I am saying that you should observe the above-mentioned precautions. By all means, stop at the first sign of chest pain. That's a basic rule under any condition; even more important when exercising in cold weather.

ALTITUDE

Another environmental factor you should take into consideration when entering an aerobics program is altitude. The 1968 Olympics in Mexico City (elevation 7300 feet above sea level) focused attention on the fact that sports and other forms of physical activity are affected by high altitude. I have received many letters from people all over the world asking if some special compensation should be made in the aerobics program when exercising at altitude.

Since the pressure of oxygen is lower at high altitude, it is obvious that performances will be impaired and some compensation must be made. The first compensation is in physical fitness testing. If a person takes a 12-minute or 1.5-mile fitness categorization test the following altitude adjustments for distance or time should be made:

12-Minute Fitness Categorization Test

Altitude in Feet at Which Acclimatized	Distances to be subtracted from the 12-Minute Age Adjusted requirements †
* 5,000	.05 miles
6,000	.06 miles
7,000	.08 miles
8,000	.10 miles
9,000	.125 miles
10,000	.150 miles
11,000	.175 miles
12,000	.20 miles

* Up to 5,000 feet, use the 12-Minute Test charts without altitude correction.

† 12-Minute Test for Men (page 30) and 12-Minute Test for Women (page 30).

1.5 MILE FITNESS CATEGORIZATION TEST

Altitude in Feet at Which Acclimatized	Times to be added to the age requirements for running 1.5 miles †
* 5,000	30 seconds
6,000	40 seconds
7,000	50 seconds
8,000	1 minute
9,000	1 min 15 sec
10,000	1 min 30 sec
11,000	1 min 45 sec
12,000	2 minutes

* Up to 5,000 feet, use the 1.5-Mile Test chart without altitude correction (page 31).

† 1.5-Mile Test for Men (page 31).

The second compensation is an adjustment in the point charts when exercising at altitude. It would be impractical to adjust all the charts so that the effect of altitude is considered but, as an example, I have revised the points for running one mile at 5000, 8000 and 12,000 feet.

POINT VALUE FOR WALKING AND RUNNING
ONE MILE AT VARIOUS ALTITUDES

1.0 Mile Standard	5,000 Feet	Points
19:59–14:30 Min	20:29–15:00	1
14:29–12:00 Min	14:59–12.30	2
11:59–10:00 Min	12:29–10:30	3
9:59– 8:00 Min	10:29– 8:30	4
7:59– 6:30 Min	8:29– 7:00 Min	5
Under 6:30 Min	Under 7:00 Min	6

8,000 Feet	12,000 Feet	Points
20:59–15:30 Min	21:29–16:30	1
15:29–13:00 Min	16:29–14:00	2
12:59–11:00 Min	13:59–12:00	3
10:59– 9:00 Min	11:59–10:00	4
8:59– 7:30 Min	9:59– 8:30	5
Under 7:30 Min	Under 8:30	6

With these compensations, the aerobics program can be used very effectively as a means of both physical fitness testing and training at altitude.

In this chapter, I have tried to give you some general advice on how to enter the aerobics program safely and effectively. But don't forget to use "common sense" in your program.

In the next chapter, we'll discuss in detail the proper way to start in the aerobics program.

6: The Age-Adjusted Exercise Charts

BEFORE STARTING INTO the aerobics program, you should classify yourself into one of two categories: either you are already in good physical condition and want to remain that way, or you are in poor condition and want to do something about it. In the first case, you are classified as a "Conditioned Beginner" and, in the second case, as an "Unconditioned Beginner." The rules for entering and proceeding through the aerobics program are different for conditioned and unconditioned people, so be certain to read the following instructions very carefully.

CONDITIONED BEGINNERS

If you have been exercising regularly, that is at least three times a week for a minimum of six weeks, and have been given the necessary medical clearance for your age (Chapter Three), you may take the 12-minute test to determine your current level of fitness.

12-MINUTE TEST
(Distances in miles covered in 12 minutes)

FITNESS CATEGORY	AGE (YEARS)			
	Under 30	*30–39*	*40–49*	*50+*
I. Very Poor	<1.0 <.95	<.95 <.85	<.85 <.75	<.80 <.65
II. Poor	1.0–1.24 .95–1.14	.95–1.14 .85–1.04	.85–1.04 .75– .94	.80– .99 .65– .84
III. Fair	1.25–1.49 1.15–1.34	1.15–1.39 1.05–1.24	1.05–1.29 .95–1.14	1.0–1.24 .85–1.04
IV. Good	1.50–1.74 1.35–1.64	1.40–1.64 1.25–1.54	1.30–1.54 1.15–1.44	1.25–1.49 1.05–1.34
V. Excellent	1.75+ 1.65+	1.65+ 1.55+	1.55+ 1.45+	1.50+ 1.35+

(The second requirement in each case is for women.)
< Means less than.

If you pass this test, reaching either category IV or V, proceed directly to page 107 and follow one of the suggested 30-point per week programs, or make up a 30-point per week program of your own from the reference charts beginning on page 111. If you failed the test, reaching only categories I, II or III, go to the instructions for "unconditioned beginners" following below.

UNCONDITIONED BEGINNERS

If you have not been exercising regularly, DO NOT take any fitness test at the start of your exercise program. Instead, begin one of the progressive, age-adjusted starter programs outlined in this chapter.

Particularly if you are over 30 and for some reason have not been able to get the kind of medical examination suggested in Chapter Three, it is absolutely essential for your safety that you begin with one of the age-adjusted *starter* programs, observing its rules strictly.

After following the starter program for *six weeks,* you have two choices:

1 You may continue the Category I program for a full 16 weeks without ever taking any fitness test at all.

2. You may want to speed up your conditioning and reach your goal in less than 16 weeks. In that case, take the 12-minute fitness test after six weeks of initial training to place yourself into one of the five fitness categories. Then proceed according to the charts for your fitness category and your age.

The charts are self-explanatory. All you need to work with them successfully is a stopwatch or a shock-resistant wristwatch with a sweep second hand. However, a few additional hints about reading the charts and setting up your exercise routine may prove helpful.

TIME GOALS

You should reach the time goals listed for each week of the conditioning program at the *end* of that particular week. Don't try to make a time goal at the beginning of the week. If you do, you may run into a snag.

People have become discouraged right at the start because they misunderstand this. For example, a man of 52, apparently in very poor condition, wrote to me: "I'm trying to follow the stationary running program. But I can't even make it for the first day. I get winded long before those 2½ minutes." Apparently he believed that it was necessary to reach the first week's goal on the first day and as a result he exceeded his endurance capacity.

He should have started his stationary running program by working out as little as 30 seconds on the first day. The next day he could have tried 60 seconds, then to 1½ minutes and so on. By the end of the first week, 2½ minutes would have been a more realistic time goal. Gradual increments are the key to the whole conditioning program. I cannot emphasize this strongly enough.

STICKING WITH IT

Let's face the facts honestly: the first six weeks are the hardest.

It takes quite a bit of push to go through the initial phase of the conditioning program. Much depends on your frame of mind. Make a firm resolution to stick with the program for eight weeks—and no weaseling out of it. Once you're past that period, I can promise you that you'll begin to enjoy your workout. After eight to ten weeks, you sense the change. You'll find yourself looking forward to your exercise, longing for it as an accustomed pleasure.

GROUP EXERCISE

If your morale needs boosting along the way, by far the sturdiest prop for sagging spirits is group exercise. It stirs your sense of competition, providing a spur as well as the reassurance of shared experience. So if you can, join an aerobics group—at least until you're over that first hurdle.

In my own neighborhood on the outskirts of San Antonio, Texas, a community aerobics group sprang up almost spontaneously. About a dozen residents started getting together every evening at a local high school track. The wives and children would come along and it soon became a family affair. Now, we have some friendly competition from time-to-time including husband-and-wife relay races. Actually any couple can join—married or not. The rules are simple. The woman starts off, running, walking, or jogging a mile as fast as she can. Then she passes the baton to her partner, who continues for another two miles. Their combined run is timed and prizes are awarded in four age-adjusted categories, based on the average age of the couple. (Women who take a few years off their age just have to run a little harder.)

To encourage beginners who are not yet in good enough shape to compete in such events, we are now planning some games and contests not based on competition with others. For example, we ask each contestant to predict the time it will take him to walk, jog, or run a certain distance. The one coming closest to his own prediction is the winner—no matter how long it takes him.

Group activities have helped many beginners get through those hard weeks at the outset by stimulating their interest and giving them moral support.

CHANGING PROGRAMS

Once you have started a conditioning program, don't switch to a different exercise until you have completed it. Your muscles become adjusted to one type of exercise and you may not be able to keep up your rate of conditioning when you go to another form of exercise. But once you have reached the 30-point-per-week level, you are free to pick any combination of activities that will add variety and pleasure to your exercise program.

PERSONAL VARIATIONS

While the eager beavers tell me the charts are too slow, others tell me they're too fast. They find it difficult to keep up with the time goals spelled out for each week.

Such cases are exceptions, but you may be one of them. It's nothing to worry about. If you find yourself trailing behind the specified rate of progress, drop back to an easier chart or just repeat the exercise program for the last week you were able to complete without trouble.

By this repetition you will build the added aerobic capacity you need to take the next step forward on the conditioning charts. If one repetition won't do it, repeat again. Eventually you'll reach the full 30-point-per-week level.

Think of it this way: it took you five, ten or maybe twenty years to get out of shape. So don't be surprised if it takes you a few extra weeks to get back into shape. I know a middle-aged businessman here in San Antonio who took 31 weeks to complete the 16-week conditioning program. More power to him! I am proud of him for sticking with it despite obvious difficulties. Now he's reaching 30 points a week and enjoying to the ultimate his newly acquired fitness.

There's no minimum rate of progress. The only really important thing is to keep earning points every week. As long as you accumulate those points, you are building aerobic capacity. You are progressing toward the goal of good cardiovascular-pulmonary fitness.

THE AEROBICS CHART PACK

1. Follow the instructions at the beginning of Chapter Six before starting into one of the following age-adjusted progressive exercise programs.

2. Then, select one of the exercise programs compatible with your age.

	YOUR PROGRAMS ARE
IF YOU ARE:	FOUND ON PAGES:
under 30 years of age	53–64
30–39 years of age	65–78
40–49 years of age	79–92
Ages 50 and older	93–106

3. When you have completed one of the age-adjusted progressive exercise programs, continue averaging at least 30 points per week, following the program of your choice.

THE 12-MINUTE TEST OF FITNESS

Do not take this test until you have complied with the instructions at the beginning of Chapter Six.

12-MINUTE TEST
(DISTANCES IN MILES)

			AGE (years)		
FITNESS CATEGORY		UNDER 30	30-39	40-49	50+
I	Very Poor	<1.0	$<.95$	$<.85$	$<.80$
II	Poor	1.0 -1.24	.95-1.14	.85-1.04	.80- .99
III	Fair	1.25-1.49	1.15-1.39	1.05-1.29	1.0 -1.24
IV	Good	1.50-1.74	1.40-1.64	1.30-1.54	1.25-1.49
V	Excellent	1.75+	1.65+	1.55+	1.50+

$<$ means less than

WALKING EXERCISE PROGRAM
(under 30 years of age)

STARTER

WEEK	DISTANCE (miles)	TIME (min)	FREQ/WK	POINTS/WK
1	1.0	15:00	5	5
2	1.0	14:00	5	10
3	1.0	13:45	5	10
4	1.5	21:30	5	15
5	1.5	21:00	5	15
6	1.5	20:30	5	15

After completing the above starter program, continue with the Category 1 conditioning program below or, if you wish to speed up your program, take the 12-minute test of fitness. If you take the test, find your category from the table at the beginning of the chart pack (page 52). If your category is I, II, or III, continue with the appropriate category below. If your category is IV or V, follow the instructions in the note at the bottom of page 54.

CONDITIONING

FITNESS CATEGORY I   (Less than 1.0 mile on 12-minute test)

WEEK	DISTANCE (miles)	TIME (min)	FREQ/WK	POINTS/WK
7	2.0	28:00	5	20
8	2.0	27:45	5	20
9	2.0	27:30	5	20
10	2.0	27:30	3	22
	and			
	2.5	33:45	2	
11	2.0	27:30	3	22
	and			
	2.5	33:30	2	
12	2.5	33:15	4	26
	and			
	3.0	41:30	1	
13	2.5	33:15	3	27
	and			
	3.0	41:15	2	
14	2.5	33:00	3	27
	and			
	3.0	40:00	2	
15	3.0	41:00	5	30
16	4.0	55:00	3	33

WALKING EXERCISE PROGRAM
(under 30 years of age)

CONDITIONING

FITNESS CATEGORY II   (1.0–1.24 miles on 12-minute test)

WEEK	DISTANCE (miles)	TIME (min)	FREQ/WK	POINTS/WK
7	2.0	27:30	5	20
8	2.0	27:30	3	22
	and			
	2.5	33:45	2	
9	2.0	27:30	3	22
	and			
	2.5	33:30	2	
10	2.5	33:15	3	27
	and			
	3.0	41:15	2	
11	2.5	33:00	3	27
	and			
	3.0	40:00	2	
12	3.0	41:00	5	30
13	4.0	55:00	3	33

FITNESS CATEGORY III   (1.25–1.49 miles on 12-minute test)

WEEK	DISTANCE (miles)	TIME (min)	FREQ/WK	POINTS/WK
7	2.5	33:15	4	26
	and			
	3.0	41:30	1	
8	2.5	33:00	3	27
	and			
	3.0	40:00	2	
9	3.0	41:00	5	30
10	4.0	55:00	3	33

After completing the progressive walking program, go to pages 107-8 and select one of the 30-point-per-week programs or develop one of your own from the point value charts beginning on page 111.

RUNNING EXERCISE PROGRAM
(under 30 years of age)

STARTER *

WEEK	DISTANCE (miles)	TIME (min)	FREQ/WK	POINTS/WK
1	1.0	13:30	5	10
2	1.0	13:00	5	10
3	1.0	12:45	5	10
4	1.0	11:45	5	15
5	1.0	11:00	5	15
6	1.0	10:30	5	15

After completing the above starter program, continue with the Category I conditioning program below or, if you wish to speed up your program, take the 12-minute test of fitness. If you take the test, find your category from the table at the beginning of the chart pack (page 52). If your category is I, II, or III, continue with the appropriate category below. If your category is IV or V, follow the instructions in the note at the bottom of page 56.

* Start the program by walking, then walk and run, or run, as necessary to meet the changing time goals.

CONDITIONING

FITNESS CATEGORY I   (Less than 1.0 mile on 12-minute test)

WEEK	DISTANCE (miles)	TIME (min)	FREQ/WK	POINTS/WK
7	1.5	18:30	5	15
8	1.5	17:30	5	15
9	1.5	16:30	4	18
10	1.0	9:30	3	21
	and			
	1.5	15:30	2	
11	1.0	8:45	3	24
	and			
	1.5	14:45	2	
12	1.0	8:30	3	24
	and			
	1.5	14:00	2	
13	1.0	8:15	3	24
	and			
	1.5	13:30	2	
14	1.0	7:55	3	27
	and			
	1.5	13:00	2	
15	1.0	7:45	2	31
	and			
	1.5	12:30	2	
	and			
	2.0	18:00	1	
16	1.5	11:55	2	32
	and			
	2.0	17:00	2	

RUNNING EXERCISE PROGRAM
(under 30 years of age)

CONDITIONING

FITNESS CATEGORY II   (1.0–1.24 miles on 12-minute test)

WEEK	DISTANCE (miles)	TIME (min)	FREQ/WK	POINTS/WK
7	1.5	17:30	5	15
8	1.5	16:30	4	18
9	1.0 and	9:30	3	21
	1.5	15:30	2	
10	1.0 and	8:45	3	24
	1.5	14:15	2	
11	1.0 and	8:15	2	26
	1.5	13:00	3	
12	1.0 and	7:45	2	31
	1.5 and	12:30	2	
	2.0	18:00	1	
13	1.5 and	11:55	2	32
	2.0	17:00	2	

FITNESS CATEGORY III   (1.25–1.49 miles on 12-minute test)

WEEK	DISTANCE (miles)	TIME (min)	FREQ/WK	POINTS/WK
7	1.5	16:30	5	22
8	1.0 and	9:00	3	24
	1.5	14:45	2	
9	1.0 and	7:55	1	32
	2.0	18:00	3	
10	1.5 and	11:55	2	32
	2.0	17:00	2	

After completing the Category I, II, or III progressive running program, go to pages 107-8 and select one of the 40-point-per-week programs or develop one of your own from the point value charts beginning on page 111.

CYCLING EXERCISE PROGRAM
(under 30 years of age)

STARTER

WEEK	DISTANCE (miles)	TIME (min)	FREQ/WK	POINTS/WK
1	2.0	10:00	5	5
2	2.0	9:00	5	5
3	2.0	7:45	5	10
4	3.0	11:50	5	15
5	3.0	11:00	5	15
6	3.0	10:30	5	15

After completing the above starter program, continue with the Category I conditioning program below or, if you wish to speed up your program, take the 12-minute test of fitness. If you take the test, find your category from the table at the beginning of the chart pack (page 52). If your category is I, II, or III, continue with the appropriate category below. If your category is IV or V, follow the instructions in the note at the bottom of page 58.

CONDITIONING

FITNESS CATEGORY I   (Less than 1.0 mile on 12-minute test)

WEEK	DISTANCE (miles)	TIME (min)	FREQ/WK	POINTS/WK
7	4.0	15:45	5	20
8	4.0	15:30	5	20
9	4.0	14:30	5	20
10	4.0	14:00	4	21
	and			
	5.0	18:30	1	
11	4.0	14:00	3	22
	and			
	5.0	18:00	2	
12	4.0	13:45	3	24
	and			
	6.0	23:30	2	
13	4.0	13:30	3	24
	and			
	6.0	23:00	2	
14	5.0	17:00	3	27
	and			
	6.0	22:00	2	
15	6.0	21:00	5	30
16	8.0	28:30	3	31½

CYCLING EXERCISE PROGRAM
(under 30 years of age)

CONDITIONING

FITNESS CATEGORY II   (1.0–1.24 miles on 12-minute test)

WEEK	DISTANCE (miles)	TIME (min)	FREQ/WK	POINTS/WK
7	4.0	14:30	5	20
8	4.0	14:00	4	21
	and			
	5.0	18:30	1	
9	4.0	14:00	3	22
	and			
	5.0	18:00	2	
10	4.0	13:30	3	24
	and			
	6.0	23:00	2	
11	5.0	17:00	3	27
	and			
	6.0	22:00	2	
12	6.0	21:00	5	30
13	8.0	28:30	3	31½

FITNESS CATEGORY III   (1.25–1.49 miles on 12-minute test)

WEEK	DISTANCE (miles)	TIME (min)	FREQ/WK	POINTS/WK
7	4.0	13:45	3	24
	and			
	6.0	23:30	2	
8	5.0	17:00	3	27
	and			
	6.0	22:00	2	
9	6.0	21:00	5	30
10	8.0	28:30	3	31½

After completing the progressive cycling program, go to pages 107-8 and select one of the 30-point-per-week programs or develop one of your own from the point value charts beginning on page 111.

SWIMMING EXERCISE PROGRAM
(under 30 years of age)

Overhand Crawl *

STARTER

WEEK	DISTANCE (yards)	TIME (min)	FREQ/WK	POINTS/WK
1	100	2:30	5	6
2	150	3:00	5	7½
3	200	4:00	5	7½
4	250	5:00	5	10
5	250	5:30	5	10
6	300	6:00	5	12½

After completing the above starter program, continue with the Category I conditioning program below or, if you wish to speed up your program, take the 12-minute test of fitness. If you take the test, find your category from the table at the beginning of the chart pack (page 52). If your category is I, II, or III, continue with the appropriate category below. If your category is IV or V, follow the instructions in the note at the bottom of page 60.

* Breaststroke is less demanding an so is backstroke. Butterfly is considerably more demanding.

CONDITIONING

FITNESS CATEGORY I   (Less than 1.0 mile on 12-minute test)

WEEK	DISTANCE (yards)	TIME (min)	FREQ/WK	POINTS/WK
7	300	6:00	5	12½
8	400	8:30	5	17½
9	400	8:30	5	17½
10	400	8:00	2	19
	and			
	500	10:30	3	
11	400	8:00	2	22
	and			
	600	12:30	3	
12	500	10:30	3	24
	and			
	700	14:30	2	
13	600	12:00	4	27½
	and			
	800	16:30	1	
14	600	11:30	3	29½
	and			
	800	16:00	2	
15	800	15:30	4	30
16	1000	19:30	3	31½

SWIMMING EXERCISE PROGRAM
(under 30 years of age)

Overhand Crawl *

CONDITIONING

FITNESS CATEGORY II   (1.0–1.24 miles on 12-minute test)

WEEK	DISTANCE (yards)	TIME (min)	FREQ/WK	POINTS/WK
7	400	8:30	5	17½
8	400	8:00	2	19
	and			
	500	10:30	3	
9	400	8:00	2	22
	and			
	600	12:30	3	
10	600	12:30	4	27¼
	and			
	800	16:30	1	
11	600	12:30	3	29½
	and			
	800	16:00	2	
12	800	15:30	4	30
13	1000	19:30	3	31½

FITNESS CATEGORY III   (1.25–1.49 miles on 12-minute test)

WEEK	DISTANCE (yards)	TIME (min)	FREQ/WK	POINTS/WK
7	500	10:30	3	24
	and			
	700	14:30	2	
8	600	12:30	3	29½
	and			
	800	16:00	2	
9	800	15:30	4	30
10	1000	19:30	3	31½

* Breaststroke is less demanding and so is backstroke. Butterfly is considerably more demanding.

After completing the progressive swimming program, go to pages 107–8 and select one of the 30-point-per-week programs or develop one of your own from the point value charts beginning on page 111.

STATIONARY RUNNING EXERCISE PROGRAM
(under 30 years of age)

STARTER

WEEK	DURATION (min)	STEPS/MIN *	FREQ/WK	POINTS/WK
1	2:30	70–80	5	4
2	5:00	70–80	5	7½
3	5:00	70–80	5	7½
4	7:30	70–80	5	11¼
5	7:30	70–80	5	11¼
6	10:00	70–80	5	15

After completing the above starter program, continue with the Category I conditioning program below or, if you wish to speed up your program, take the 12-minute test of fitness. If you take the test, find your category from the table at the beginning of the chart pack (page 52). If your category is I, II, or III, continue with the appropriate category below. If your category is IV or V, follow the instructions in the note at the bottom of page 62.

* Count only when the left foot hits the floor. Feet must be brought at least eight inches from the floor.

CONDITIONING

FITNESS CATEGORY I   (Less than 1.0 mile on 12-minute test)

WEEK	DURATION (min)	STEPS/MIN *	FREQ/WK	POINTS/WK
7	10:00	70–80	5	15
8	12:30	70–80	5	18¾
9	12:30	70–80	5	18¾
10	15:00	70–80	5	22½
11	15:00	70–80	5	22½
12	10:00	80–90	1	24¼
	and			
	17:30	70–80	3	
13	12:30	80–90	3	27
	and			
	15:00	80–90	2	
14	12:30	80–90	2	28
	and			
	15:00	80–90	3	
15	15:00	80–90	5	30
16	15:00	90–100	4	30

* Count only when the left foot hits the floor. Feet must be brought at least eight inches from the floor.

STATIONARY RUNNING EXERCISE PROGRAM
(under 30 years of age)

CONDITIONING

FITNESS CATEGORY II   (1.0–1.24 miles on 12-minute test)

WEEK	DURATION (min)	STEPS/MIN *	FREQ/WK	POINTS/WK
7	12:30	70–80	5	18¾
8	15:00	70–80	5	22½
9	15:00	70–80	5	22½
10	12:30	80–90	3	27
	and			
	15:00	80–90	2	
11	12:30	80–90	2	28
	and			
	15:00	80–90	3	
12	15:00	80–90	5	30
13	15:00	90–100	4	30

* Count only when the left foot hits the floor. Feet must be brought at least eight inches from the floor.

FITNESS CATEGORY III   (1.25–1.49 miles on 12-minute test)

WEEK	DURATION (min)	STEPS/MIN *	FREQ/WK	POINTS/WK
7	10:00	80–90	1	24¼
	and			
	17:30	70–80	3	
8	12:30	80–90	2	28
	and			
	15:00	80–90	3	
9	15:00	80–90	5	30
10	15:00	90–100	4	30

* Count only when the left foot hits the floor. Feet must be brought at least eight inches from the floor.

After completing the progressive program, go to pages 107-8 and select one of the 30-point-per-week programs or develop one of your own from the point value charts beginning on page 111.

HANDBALL/BASKETBALL/SQUASH EXERCISE PROGRAM
(under 30 years of age)

STARTER

WEEK	TIME (min)*	FREQ/WK	POINTS/WK
1	10	5	7½
2	15	5	11¼
3	15	5	11¼
4	20	5	15
5	20	5	15
6	20	5	15

After completing the above starter program, continue with the Category I conditioning program below or, if you wish to speed up your program, take the 12-minute test of fitness. If you take the test, find your category from the table at the beginning of the chart pack (page 52). If your category is I, II, or III, continue with the appropriate category below. If your category is IV or V, follow the instructions in the note at the bottom of page 64.

* Continuous exercise. Do not count breaks, time-outs, etc.

CONDITIONING

FITNESS CATEGORY I   (Less than 1.0 mile on 12-minute test)

WEEK	TIME (min)*	FREQ/WK	POINTS/WK
7	30	5	22½
8	30	5	22½
9	30	5	22½
10	35	5	26¼
11	35	5	26¼
12	35 and 40	3 2	27¼
13	35 and 40	3 2	27¼
14	30 and 45	2 3	29¼
15	40	5	30
16	50	4	30

* Continuous exercise. Do not count breaks, time-outs, etc.

HANDBALL/BASKETBALL/SQUASH EXERCISE PROGRAM
(under 30 years of age)

CONDITIONING

FITNESS CATEGORY II   (1.0–1.24 miles on the 12-minute test)

WEEK	TIME (min) *	FREQ/WK	POINTS/WK
7	30	5	22½
8	35	5	26¼
9	35	5	26¼
10	35	3	27¼
	and		
	40	2	
11	30	2	29¼
	and		
	45	3	
12	40	5	30
13	50	4	30

* Continuous exercise. Do not count breaks, time-outs, etc.

FITNESS CATEGORY III   (1.25–1.49 miles on the 12-minute test)

WEEK	TIME (min) *	FREQ/WK	POINTS/WK
7	35	3	27¼
	and		
	40	2	
8	30	2	29¼
	and		
	45	3	
9	40	5	30
10	50	4	30

* Continuous exercise. Do not count breaks, time-outs, etc.

After completing the progressive program, go to pages 107-8 and select one of the 30-point-per-week programs or develop one of your own from the point value charts beginning on page 111.

WALKING EXERCISE PROGRAM
(30–39 years of age)

STARTER

WEEK	DISTANCE (miles)	TIME (min)	FREQ/WK	POINTS/WK
1	1.0	17:30	5	5
2	1.0	15:30	5	5
3	1.0	14:15	5	10
4	1.0	14:00	5	10
5	1.5	21:40	5	15
6	1.5	21:15	5	15

After completing the above starter program, continue with the Category I conditioning program below, or if you wish to speed up your program, take the 12-minute test of fitness. If you take the test, find your category from the table at the beginning of the chart pack (page 52). If your category is I, II, or III, continue with the appropriate category below. If your category is IV or V, follow the instructions in the note at the bottom of page 66.

CONDITIONING

FITNESS CATEGORY I   (Less than 0.95 mile on 12-minute test)

WEEK	DISTANCE (miles)	TIME (min)	FREQ/WK	POINTS/WK
7	1.5	21:00	5	15
8	2.0	28:45	5	20
9	2.0	28:30	5	20
10	2.0	28:00	5	20
11	2.0	28:00	3	22
	and			
	2.5	35:30	2	
12	2.5	35:00	3	27
	and			
	3.0	43:15	2	
13	2.5	34:45	3	27
	and			
	3.0	43:00	2	
14	2.5	34:30	3	27
	and			
	3.0	42:30	2	
15	3.0	42:30	5	30
16	4.0	56:30	3	33

WALKING EXERCISE PROGRAM
(30–39 years of age)

CONDITIONING

FITNESS CATEGORY II   (0.95–1.14 miles on 12-minute test)

WEEK	DISTANCE (miles)	TIME (min)	FREQ/WK	POINTS/WK
7	2.0	28:30	5	20
8	2.0	28:00	5	20
9	2.0	28:00	3	22
	and			
	2.5	35:30	2	
10	2.5	34:45	3	27
	and			
	3.0	43:00	2	
11	2.5	34:30	3	27
	and			
	3.0	42:30	2	
12	3.0	42:30	5	30
13	4.0	56:30	3	33

FITNESS CATEGORY III   (1.15–1.39 miles on 12-minute test)

WEEK	DISTANCE (miles)	TIME (min)	FREQ/WK	POINTS/WK
7	2.5	35:00	3	27
	and			
	3.0	43:15	2	
8	2.5	34:30	3	27
	and			
	3.0	42:30	2	
9	3.0	42:30	5	30
10	4.0	56:30	3	33

After completing the Category I, II, or III progressive running program, go to pages 107–8 and select one of the 30-point-per-week programs or develop one of your own from the point value charts beginning on page 111.

RUNNING EXERCISE PROGRAM
(30–39 years of age)

STARTER *

WEEK	DISTANCE (miles)	TIME (min)	FREQ/WK	POINTS/WK
1	1.0	17:30	5	5
2	1.0	15:30	5	5
3	1.0	14:15	5	10
4	1.0	13:30	5	10
5	1.0	11:45	5	15
6	1.0	11:15	5	15

After completing the above starter program, continue with the Category I conditioning program below or, if you wish to speed up your program, take the 12-minute test of fitness. If you take the test, find your category from the table at the beginning of the chart pack (page 52). If your category is I, II, or III, continue with the appropriate category below. If your category is IV or V, follow the instructions in the note at the bottom of page 70.

* Start the program by walking. Then walk and run, or run, as necessary to meet the changing time goals.

RUNNING EXERCISE PROGRAM
(30–39 years of age)

CONDITIONING

FITNESS CATEGORY I   (Less than 0.95 mile on 12-minute test)

WEEK	DISTANCE (miles)	TIME (min)	FREQ/WK	POINTS/WK
7	1.5	19:30	5	15
8	1.5	18:30	5	15
9	1.5	17:30	4	18
10	1.0 and	10:00	2	19½
	1.5	16:30	3	
11	1.0 and	9:30	3	21
	1.5	15:30	2	
12	1.0 and	9:00	3	24
	1.5	14:30	2	
13	1.0 and	8:30	3	24
	1.5	14:00	2	
14	1.0 and	8:15	3	30
	2.0	19:30	2	
15	1.0 and	8:00	2	31½
	1.5 and	12:55	2	
	2.5	22:30	1	
16	1.0 and	8:00	1	34
	1.5 and	12:25	2	
	2.0	18:30	2	

RUNNING EXERCISE PROGRAM
(30–39 years of age)

CONDITIONING

FITNESS CATEGORY II   (0.95–1.14 miles on 12-minute test)

WEEK	DISTANCE (miles)	TIME (min)	FREQ/WK	POINTS/WK
7	1.5	18:30	5	15
8	1.5	17:00	4	18
9	1.0	10:00	3	21
	and			
	1.5	15:45	2	
10	1.0	9:15	3	24
	and			
	1.5	14:30	2	
11	1.0	8:45	2	26
	and			
	1.5	13:00	3	
12	1.0	8:15	3	30
	and			
	2.0	19:30	2	
13	1.0	8:00	1	34
	and			
	1.5	12:25	2	
	and			
	2.0	18:30	2	

RUNNING EXERCISE PROGRAM
(30–39 years of age)

CONDITIONING

FITNESS CATEGORY III   (1.15–1.39 miles on 12-minute test)

WEEK	DISTANCE (miles)	TIME (min)	FREQ/WK	POINTS/WK
7	1.5	17:30	4	18
8	1.0	10:00	1	21
	and			
	1.5	15:15	4	
9	1.5	13:15	3	27
	and			
	2.0	19:30	1	
10	1.0	8:00	1	34
	and			
	1.5	12:25	2	
	and			
	2.0	18:30	2	

After completing the Category I, II, or III progressive running program, go to pages 107–8 and select one of the 30-point-per-week programs or develop one of your own from the point value charts beginning on page 111.

CYCLING EXERCISE PROGRAM
(30–39 years of age)

STARTER

WEEK	DISTANCE (miles)	TIME (min)	FREQ/WK	POINTS/WK
1	2	10:30	5	5
2	2	9:30	5	5
3	2	8:30	5	5
4	2	7:45	5	10
5	2	7:30	5	10
6	3	11:50	5	15

After completing the above starter program, continue with the Category I conditioning program below or, if you wish to speed up your program, take the 12-minute test of fitness. If you take the test, find your category from the table at the beginning of the chart pack (page 52). If your category is I, II, or III, continue with the appropriate category below. If your category is IV or V, follow the instructions in the note at the bottom of page 72.

CONDITIONING

FITNESS CATEGORY I   (Less than 0.95 mile on 12-minute test)

WEEK	DISTANCE (miles)	TIME (min)	FREQ/WK	POINTS/WK
7	3.0	11:30	5	15
8	4.0	15:45	5	20
9	4.0 and	15:30	4	21
	5.0	19:45	1	
10	4.0 and	15:00	3	22
	5.0	19:00	2	
11	3.0 and	11:00	2	24
	6.0	23:45	3	
12	3.0 and	10:30	2	24
	6.0	23:30	3	
13	3.0 and	10:30	2	24
	6.0	23:00	3	
14	5.0 and	18:30	3	27
	6.0	22:30	2	
15	6.0	22:00	5	30
16	8.0	29:30	3	31½

CYCLING EXERCISE PROGRAM
(30–39 years of age)

CONDITIONING

FITNESS CATEGORY II   (0.95–1.14 miles on 12-minute test)

WEEK	DISTANCE (miles)	TIME (min)	FREQ/WK	POINTS/WK
7	4.0	15:30	4	21
	and			
	5.0	19:45	1	
8	4.0	15:00	3	22
	and			
	5.0	19:00	2	
9	3.0	11:00	2	24
	and			
	6.0	23:45	3	
10	3.0	10:30	2	24
	and			
	6.0	23:00	3	
11	5.0	18:30	3	27
	and			
	6.0	22:30	2	
12	6.0	22:00	5	30
13	8.0	29:30	3	31½

FITNESS CATEGORY III   (1.15–1.39 miles on 12-minute test)

WEEK	DISTANCE (miles)	TIME (min)	FREQ/WK	POINTS/WK
7	3.0	10:30	2	24
	and			
	6.0	23:30	3	
8	5.0	18:30	3	27
	and			
	6.0	22:30	2	
9	6.0	22:00	5	30
10	8.0	29:30	3	31½

After completing the Category I, II, or III progressive cycling program, go to pages 107–8 and select one of the 30-point-per-week programs or develop one of your own from the point value charts beginning on page 111.

SWIMMING EXERCISE PROGRAM
(30–39 years of age)

Overhand Crawl *

STARTER

WEEK	DISTANCE (yards)	TIME (min)	FREQ/WK	POINTS/WK
1	100	2:30	5	4
2	150	3:00	5	5
3	175	3:45	5	6
4	200	4:00	5	7½
5	250	5:15	5	10
6	250	5:00	5	10

After completing the above starter program, continue with the Category I conditioning program below or, if you wish to speed up your program, take the 12-minute test of fitness. If you take the test, find your category from the table at the beginning of the chart pack (page 52). If your Category is I, II, or III, continue with the appropriate category below. If your category is IV or V, follow the instructions in the note at the bottom of page 74.

* Breaststroke is less demanding and so is backstroke. Butterfly is considerably more demanding.

CONDITIONING

FITNESS CATEGORY I   (Less than 0.95 mile on 12-minute test)

WEEK	DISTANCE (yards)	TIME (min)	FREQ/WK	POINTS/WK
7	300	6.15	5	12½
8	300	6:00	5	12½
9	400	8:30	5	17½
10	400	8:00	5	17½
11	400	8:00	2	19
	and			
	500	10:30	3	
12	400	8:30	2	22
	and			
	600	12:30	3	
13	500	10:30	3	24
	and			
	700	15:00	2	
14	600	12:00	4	27¼
	and			
	800	16:30	1	
15	800	16:00	4	30
16	1000	20:30	3	31½

SWIMMING EXERCISE PROGRAM
(30–39 years of age)

Overhand Crawl *

FITNESS CATEGORY II   (0.95–1.14 miles on 12-minute test)

WEEK	DISTANCE (yards)	TIME (min)	FREQ/WK	POINTS/WK
7	400	8:30	5	17½
8	400	8:00	5	17½
9	400	8:00	2	19
	and			
	500	10:30	3	
10	500	10:30	3	24
	and			
	700	15:00	2	
11	600	12:00	4	27¼
	and			
	800	16:30	1	
12	800	16:00	4	30
13	1000	20:30	3	31½

FITNESS CATEGORY III   (1.15–1.39 miles on 12-minute test)

WEEK	DISTANCE (yards)	TIME (min)	FREQ/WK	POINTS/WK
7	400	8:30	2	22
	and			
	600	12:30	3	
8	600	12:00	4	27¼
	and			
	800	16:30	1	
9	800	16:00	4	30
10	1000	20:30	3	31½

* Breaststroke is less demanding and so is backstoke. Butterfly is considerably more demanding.

After completing the Category I, II, or III progressive swimming program, go to pages 107–8 and select one of the 30-point-per-week programs or develop one of your own from the point value charts beginning on page 111.

STATIONARY RUNNING EXERCISE PROGRAM
(30–39 years of age)

STARTER

WEEK	DURATION (min)	STEPS/MIN *	FREQ/WK	POINTS/WK
1	2:30	70–80	5	4
2	2:30	70–80	5	4
3	5:00	70–80	5	7½
4	5:00	70–80	5	7½
5	7:30	70–80	5	11¼
6	7:30	70–80	5	11¼

After completing the above starter program, continue with the Category I conditioning program below or, if you wish to speed up your program, take the 12-minute test of fitness. If you take the test, find your category from the table at the beginning of the chart pack (page 52). If your category is I, II, or III, continue with the appropriate category below. If your category is IV or V, follow the instructions in the note at the bottom of page 76.

* Count only when the left foot hits the floor. Feet must be brought at least eight inches from the floor.

CONDITIONING

FITNESS CATEGORY I   (Less than 0.95 mile on 12-minute test)

WEEK	DURATION (min)	STEPS/MIN *	FREQ/WK	POINTS/WK
7	10:00	70–80	5	15
8	10:00	70–80	5	15
9	12:30	70–80	5	18¾
10	12:30	70–80	5	18¾
11	15:00	70–80	5	22½
12	10:00 and	80–90	1	24¼
	17:30	70–80	3	
13	10:00 and	80–90	1	24¼
	17:30	70–80	3	
14	12:30 and	80–90	2	28
	15:00	80–90	3	
15	15:00	80–90	5	30
16	15:00	90–100	4	30

* Count only when the left foot hits the floor. Feet must be brought at least eight inches from the floor.

STATIONARY RUNNING EXERCISE PROGRAM
(30–39 years of age)

CONDITIONING

FITNESS CATEGORY II   (0.95–1.4 miles on 12-minute test)

WEEK	DURATION (min)	STEPS/MIN *	FREQ/WK	POINTS/WK
7	12:30	70–80	5	18¾
8	12:30	70–80	5	18¾
9	15:00	70–80	5	22½
10	10:00	80–90	1	24¼
	and			
	17:30	70–80	3	
11	12:30	80–90	2	28
	and			
	15:00	80–90	3	
12	15:00	80–90	5	30
13	15:00	90–100	4	30

* Count only when the left foot hits the floor. Feet must be brought at least eight inches from the floor.

FITNESS CATEGORY III   (1.15–1.39 miles on 12-minute test)

WEEK	DURATION (min)	STEPS/MIN *	FREQ/WK	POINTS/WK
7	10:00	80–90	1	24¼
	and			
	17:30	70–80	3	
8	12:30	80–90	2	28
	and			
	15:00	80–90	3	
9	15:00	80–90	5	30
10	15:00	90–100	4	30

* Count only when the left foot hits the floor. Feet must be brought at least eight inches from the floor.

After completing the Category I, II, or III progressive stationary running program, go to pages 107–8 and select one of the 30-point-per-week programs or develop one of your own from the point value charts beginning on page 111.

HANDBALL/BASKETBALL/SQUASH EXERCISE PROGRAM
(30–39 years of age)

STARTER

WEEK	TIME(min)*	FREQ/WK	POINTS/WK
1	10	5	7½
2	10	5	7½
3	15	5	11¼
4	15	5	11¼
5	20	5	15
6	20	5	15

After completing the above starter program, continue with the Category I conditioning program below or, if you wish to speed up your program, take the 12-minute test of fitness. If you take the test, find your category from the table at the beginning of the chart pack (page 52). If your category is I, II, or III, continue with the appropriate category below. If your category is IV or V, follow the instructions in the note at the bottom of page 78.

* Continuous exercise. Do not count breaks, time-outs, etc.

CONDITIONING

FITNESS CATEGORY I   (Less than 0.95 mile on 12-minute test)

WEEK	TIME(min)*	FREQ/WK	POINTS/WK
7	20	5	15
8	25	5	18¾
9	20	1	21
	and		
	30	4	
10	20	1	21
	and		
	30	4	
11	25	1	24¾
	and		
	35	4	
12	25	1	24¾
	and		
	35	4	
13	35	3	27¾
	and		
	40	2	
14	35	3	27¾
	and		
	40	2	
15	40	5	30
16	50	4	30

* Continuous exercise. Do not count breaks, time-outs, etc.

90222

HANDBALL/BASKETBALL/SQUASH EXERCISE PROGRAM
(30–39 years of age)

CONDITIONING

FITNESS CATEGORY II   (0.95–1.14 miles on 12-minute test)

WEEK	TIME (min)*	FREQ/WK	POINTS/WK
7	20	1	21
	and		
	30	4	
8	20	1	21
	and		
	30	4	
9	25	1	24¾
	and		
	35	4	
10	35	3	27¾
	and		
	40	2	
11	35	3	27¾
	and		
	40	2	
12	40	5	30
13	50	4	30

* Continuous exercise. Do not count breaks, time-outs, etc.

FITNESS CATEGORY III   (1.15–1.39 miles on 12-minute test)

WEEK	TIME (min)*	FREQ/WK	POINTS/WK
7	25	1	24¾
	and		
	35	4	
8	35	3	27¾
	and		
	40	2	
9	40	5	30
10	50	4	30

* Continuous exercise. Do not count breaks, time-outs, etc.

After completing the Category I, II, or III progressive program, go to pages 107–8 and select one of the 30-point-per-week programs or develop one of your own from the point value charts beginning on page 111.

WALKING EXERCISE PROGRAM
(40–49 years of age)

STARTER

WEEK	DISTANCE (miles)	TIME (min)	FREQ/WK	POINTS/WK
1	1.0	18:00	5	5
2	1.0	16:00	5	5
3	1.5	24:00	5	7½
4	1.5	22:30	5	7½
5	2.0	31:00	5	10
6	2.0	30:00	5	10

After completing the above starter program, continue with the Category I conditioning program below or, if you wish to speed up your program, take the 12-minute test of fitness. If you take the test, find your category from the table at the beginning of the chart pack (page 52). If your category is I, II, or III, continue with the appropriate category below. If your category is IV or V, follow the instructions in the note at the bottom of page 80.

CONDITIONING

FITNESS CATEGORY I   (Less than 0.85 mile on 12-minute test)

WEEK	DISTANCE (miles)	TIME (min)	FREQ/WK	POINTS/WK
7	2.5	37:45	5	12½
8	2.5	36:30	5	12½
9	2.0 and	29:30	3	16
	2.5	36:00	2	
10	1.5 and	21:30	3	19
	2.5	35:30	2	
11	2.0 and	28:00	3	22
	2.5	36:00	2	
12	2.5 and	35:30	4	23
	3.0	43:45	1	
13	2.0 and	28:00	2	26
	3.0	43:00	3	
14	2.5 and	34:45	3	27
	3.0	42:45	2	
15	3.0	42:45	5	30
16	4.0	56:45	3	33

WALKING EXERCISE PROGRAM
(40–49 years of age)

CONDITIONING

FITNESS CATEGORY II   (0.85–1.04 miles on 12-minute test)

WEEK	DISTANCE (miles)	TIME (min)	FREQ/WK	POINTS/WK
7	2.0	29:30	3	16
	and			
	2.5	36:00	2	
8	1.5	21:30	3	19
	and			
	2.5	35:30	2	
9	2.0	28:00	3	22
	and			
	2.5	36:00	2	
10	2.0	28:00	2	26
	and			
	3.0	43:00	3	
11	2.5	34:45	3	27
	and			
	3.0	42:45	2	
12	3.0	42:45	5	30
13	4.0	56:45	3	33

FITNESS CATEGORY III   (1.05–1.29 miles on 12-minute test)

WEEK	DISTANCE (miles)	TIME (min)	FREQ/WK	POINTS/WK
7	2.5	35:30	4	23
	and			
	3.0	43:45	1	
8	2.5	34:45	3	27
	and			
	3.0	42:45	2	
9	3.0	42:45	5	30
10	4.0	56:45	3	33

After completing the Category I, II, or III progressive walking program, go to pages 107–8 and select one of the 30-point-per-week programs or develop one of your own from the point value charts beginning on page 111.

RUNNING EXERCISE PROGRAM
(40–49 years of age)

STARTER *

WEEK	DISTANCE (miles)	TIME (min)	FREQ/WK	POINTS/WK
1	1.0	18:00	5	5
2	1.0	16:00	5	5
3	1.0	15:00	5	5
4	1.0	14:15	5	10
5	1.0	13:45	5	10
6	1.0	12:45	5	10

After completing the above starter program, continue with the Category I conditioning program below or, if you wish to speed up your program, take the 12-minute test of fitness. If you take the test, find your category from the table at the beginning of the chart pack (page 52). If your category is I, II, or III, continue with the appropriate category below. If your category is IV or V, follow the instructions in the note at the bottom of page 84.

* Start the program by walking, then walk and run, or run as necessary to meet the changing time goals.

RUNNING EXERCISE PROGRAM
(40–49 years of age)

CONDITIONING

FITNESS CATEGORY I   (Less than 0.85 mile on 12-minute test)

WEEK	DISTANCE (miles)	TIME (min)	FREQ/WK	POINTS/WK
7	1.5	20:30	5	15
8	1.5	19:30	5	15
9	1.5	18:30	5	15
10	1.0	10:45	2	19½
	and			
	1.5	17:30	3	
11	1.0	10:15	2	19½
	and			
	1.5	16:30	3	
12	1.0	9:45	3	21
	and			
	1.5	15:30	2	
13	1.0	9:15	3	24
	and			
	1.5	14:55	2	
14	1.0	8:55	3	26
	and			
	2.0	20:30	2	
15	1.0	8:45	2	27
	and			
	1.5	14:00	2	
	and			
	2.0	20:00	1	
16	1.0	8:30	1	34
	and			
	1.5	13:25	2	
	and			
	2.0	19:30	2	

RUNNING EXERCISE PROGRAM
(40–49 years of age)

CONDITIONING

FITNESS CATEGORY II   (0.85–1.04 miles on 12-minute test)

WEEK	DISTANCE (miles)	TIME (min)	FREQ/WK	POINTS/WK
7	1.5	19:30	5	15
8	1.5	18:00	5	15
9	1.0	10:45	3	18
	and			
	1.5	17:00	2	
10	1.0	10:00	1	21
	and			
	1.5	15:45	4	
11	1.0	9:30	2	26
	and			
	1.5	14:30	3	
12	1.0	9:00	1	32
	and			
	2.0	20:30	4	
13	1.0	8:30	1	34
	and			
	1.5	13:25	2	
	and			
	2.0	19:30	2	

RUNNING EXERCISE PROGRAM
(40–49 years of age)

CONDITIONING

FITNESS CATEGORY III   (1.05–1.29 miles on 12-minute test)

WEEK	DISTANCE (miles)	TIME (min)	FREQ/WK	POINTS/WK
7	1.5	18:30	5	15
8	1.0	10:45	3	18
	and			
	1.5	16:30	2	
9	1.5	14:15	2	26
	and			
	2.0	20:30	2	
10	1.0	8:30	1	34
	and			
	1.5	13:25	2	
	and			
	2.0	19:30	2	

After completing the Category I, II, or III progressive running program, go to pages 107–8 and select one of the 30-point-per-week program or develop one of your own from the point value charts beginning on page 111.

CYCLING EXERCISE PROGRAM
(40–49 years of age)

STARTER

WEEK	DISTANCE (miles)	TIME (min)	FREQ/WK	POINTS/WK
1	2.0	11:00	5	5
2	2.0	10:00	5	5
3	3.0	15:00	5	7½
4	3.0	14:00	5	7½
5	4.0	19:00	5	10
6	4.0	17:30	5	10

After completing the above starter program, continue with the Category I conditioning program below or, if you wish to speed up your program, take the 12-minute test of fitness. If you take the test, find your category from the table at the beginning of the chart pack (page 52). If your category is I, II, or III, continue with the appropriate category below. If your category is IV or V, follow the instructions in the note at the bottom of page 86.

CONDITIONING

FITNESS CATEGORY I   (Less than 0.85 mile on 12-minute test)

WEEK	DISTANCE (miles)	TIME (min)	FREQ/WK	POINTS/WK
7	4.0	16:30	5	10
8	5.0	21:30	5	12½
9	3.0 and	13:00	2	15
	4.0	15:45	3	
10	3.0 and	11:45	1	18
	4.0	15:30	4	
11	4.0 and	15:00	3	22
	5.0	19:45	2	
12	3.0 and	11:30	2	24
	6.0	23:45	3	
13	3.0 and	11:00	2	24
	6.0	23:30	3	
14	5.0 and	19:00	3	27
	6.0	23:15	2	
15	6.0	23:00	5	30
16	8.0	31:30	3	31½

CYCLING EXERCISE PROGRAM
(40–49 years of age)

CONDITIONING

FITNESS CATEGORY II   (0.85–1.04 miles on 12-minute test)

WEEK	DISTANCE (miles)	TIME (min)	FREQ/WK	POINTS/WK
7	3.0	13:00	2	15
	and			
	4.0	15:45	3	
8	3.0	11:45	1	18
	and			
	4.0	15:30	4	
9	4.0	15:00	3	22
	and			
	5.0	19:45	2	
10	3.0	11:00	2	24
	and			
	6.0	23:30	3	
11	5.0	19:00	3	27
	and			
	6.0	23:15	2	
12	6.0	23:00	5	30
13	8.0	31:30	3	31½

FITNESS CATEGORY III   (1.05–1.29 miles on 12-minute test)

WEEK	DISTANCE (miles)	TIME (min)	FREQ/WK	POINTS/WK
7	3.0	11:30	2	24
	and			
	6.0	23:45	3	
8	5.0	19:00	3	27
	and			
	6.0	23:15	2	
9	6.0	23:00	5	30
10	8.0	31:30	3	31½

After completing the Category I, II, or III progressive cycling program, go to pages 107–8 and select one of the 30-point-per-week programs or develop one of your own from the point value charts beginning on page 111.

SWIMMING EXERCISE PROGRAM
(40–49 years of age)

Overhand Crawl *

STARTER

WEEK	DISTANCE (yards)	TIME (min)	FREQ/WK	POINTS/WK
1	100	2:30	5	4
2	150	3:15	5	5
3	175	4:00	5	6
4	200	4:30	5	7½
5	200	4:15	5	7½
6	250	5:30	5	10

After completing the above starter program, continue with the Category I conditioning program below or, if you wish to speed up your program, take the 12-minute test of fitness. If you take the test, find your category from the table at the beginning of the chart pack (page 52). If your category is I, II, or III, continue with the appropriate category below. If your category is IV or V, follow the instructions in the note at the bottom of page 88.

* Breaststroke is less demanding and so is backstroke. Butterfly is considerably more demanding.

CONDITIONING

FITNESS CATEGORY I   (Less than 0.85 mile on 12-minute test)

WEEK	DISTANCE (yards)	TIME (min)	FREQ/WK	POINTS/WK
7	250	5:15	5	10
8	300	6:45	5	12½
9	300	6:15	5	12½
10	400	9:00	5	17½
11	400	8:30	5	17½
12	400	8:30	2	19
	and			
	500	10:45	3	
13	400	9:00	2	22
	and			
	600	13:00	3	
14	500	11:00	3	24
	and			
	700	15:30	2	
15	700	15:00	5	30
16	800	16:30	4	30

SWIMMING EXERCISE PROGRAM
(40–49 years of age)

Overhand Crawl *

CONDITIONING

FITNESS CATEGORY II   (0.85–1.04 miles on 12-minute test)

WEEK	DISTANCE (yards)	TIME (min)	FREQ/WK	POINTS/WK
7	300	6:15	5	12½
8	400	9:00	5	17½
9	400	8:30	5	17½
10	400 and	9:00	2	22
	600	13:00	3	
11	500 and	11:00	3	24
	700	15:30	2	
12	700	15:00	5	30
13	800	16:30	4	30

FITNESS CATEGORY III   (1.05–1.29 miles on 12-minute test)

WEEK	DISTANCE (yards)	TIME (min)	FREQ/WK	POINTS/WK
7	400 and	8:30	2	19
	500	10:45	3	
8	500 and	11:00	3	24
	700	15:30	2	
9	700	15:00	5	30
10	800	16:30	4	30

* Breaststroke is less demanding and so is backstroke. Butterfly is considerably more demanding.

After completing the Category I, II, or III progressive swimming program, go to pages 107–8 and select one of the 30-point-per-week programs or develop one of your own from the point value charts beginning on page 111.

STATIONARY RUNNING EXERCISE PROGRAM
(40–49 years of age)

STARTER

WEEK	DURATION (min)	STEPS/MIN *	FREQ/WK	POINTS/WK
1	2:30	70–80	5	4
2	2:30	70–80	5	4
3	5:00	70–80	5	7½
4	5:00	70–80	5	7½
5	5:00	70–80	5	7½
6	7:30	70–80	5	11¼

After completing the above starter program, continue with the Category I conditioning program below or, if you wish to speed up your program, take the 12-minute test of fitness. If you take the test, find your category from the table at the beginning of the chart pack (page 52). If your category is I, II, or III, continue with the appropriate category below. If your category is IV or V, follow the instructions in the note at the bottom of page 90.

* Count only when the left foot strikes the floor. Feet must be brought at least eight inches from the floor.

CONDITIONING

FITNESS CATEGORY I   (Less than 0.85 mile on 12-minute test)

WEEK	DURATION (min)	STEPS/MIN *	FREQ/WK	POINTS/WK
7	7:30	70–80	5	11¼
8	10:00	70–80	5	15
9	10:00	70–80	5	15
10	12:30	70–80	5	18¾
11	12:30	70–80	5	18¾
12	15:00	70–80	5	22½
13	10:00 and	80–90	1	24¼
	17:30	70–80	3	
14	12:30 and	80–90	2	28
	15:00	80–90	3	
15	17:30	70–80	4	27
16	20:00	80–90	3	30

* Count only when the left foot strikes the floor. Feet must be brought at least eight inches from the floor.

STATIONARY RUNNING EXERCISE PROGRAM
(40–49 years of age)

CONDITIONING

FITNESS CATEGORY II   (0.85–1.04 miles on 12-minute test)

WEEK	DURATION (min)	STEPS/MIN *	FREQ/WK	POINTS/WK
7	10:00	70–80	5	15
8	12:30	70–80	5	18¾
9	12:30	70–80	5	18¾
10	10:00	80–90	1	24¼
	and			
	17:30	70–80	3	
11	12:30	80–90	2	28
	and			
	15:00	80–90	3	
12	17:30	70–80	4	27
13	20:00	80–90	3	30

* Count only when the left foot strikes the floor. Feet must be brought at least eight inches from the floor.

FITNESS CATEGORY III   (1.05–1.29 miles on 12-minute test)

WEEK	DURATION (min)	STEPS/MIN *	FREQ/WK	POINTS/WK
7	15:00	70–80	5	22½
8	12:30	80–90	2	28
	and			
	15:00	80–90	3	
9	17:30	70–80	4	27
10	20:00	80–90	3	30

* Count only when the left foot strikes the floor. Feet must be brought at least eight inches from the floor.

After completing the Category I, II, or III progressive stationary running program, go to pages 107–8 and select one of the 30-point-per-week programs or develop one of your own from the point value charts beginning on page 111.

HANDBALL/BASKETBALL/SQUASH EXERCISE PROGRAM
(40–49 years af age)

STARTER

WEEK	TIME (min) *	FREQ/WK	POINTS/WK
1	10	5	7½
2	10	5	7½
3	10	5	7½
4	15	5	11¼
5	15	5	11¼
6	15	5	11¼

After completing the above starter program, continue with the Category I conditioning program below or if, you wish to speed up your program, take the 12-minute test of fitness. If you take the test, find your category from the table at the beginning of the chart pack (page 52). If your category is I, II, or III, continue with the appropriate category below. If your category is IV or V, follow the instructions in the note at the bottom of page 92.

* Continuous exercise. Do not count breaks, time-outs, etc.

CONDITIONING

Fitness Category I   (Less than 0.85 mile on 12-minute test)

WEEK	TIME (min) *	FREQ/WK	POINTS/WK
7	20	5	15
8	20	5	15
9	20	5	15
10	25	5	18¾
11	25	5	18¾
12	20	1	21
	and		
	30	4	
13	20	1	21
	and		
	30	4	
14	25	1	24¾
	and		
	35	4	
15	35	3	27¾
	and		
	40	2	
16	40	5	30

* Continuous exercise. Do not count breaks, time-outs, etc.

HANDBALL/BASKETBALL/SQUASH EXERCISE PROGRAM
(40–49 years af age)

CONDITIONING

FITNESS CATEGORY II   (0.85–1.04 miles on 12-minute test)

WEEK	TIME (min) *	FREQ/WK	POINTS/WK
7	20	5	15
8	25	5	18¾
9	25	5	18¾
10	20	1	21
	and		
	30	4	
11	25	1	24¾
	and		
	35	4	
12	35	3	27¾
	and		
	40	2	
13	40	5	30

* Continuous exercise. Do not count breaks, time-outs, etc.

FITNESS CATEGORY III   (1.05–1.29 miles on 12-minute test)

WEEK	TIME (min) *	FREQ/WK	POINTS/WK
7	20	1	21
	and		
	30	4	
8	25	1	24¾
	and		
	35	4	
9	35	3	27¾
	and		
	40	2	
10	40	5	30

* Continuous exercise. Do not count breaks, time-outs, etc.

After completing the Category I, II, or III progressive program, go to pages 107–8 and select one of the 30-point-per-week programs or develop one of your own from the point value charts beginning on page 111.

WALKING EXERCISE PROGRAM
(age 50 and over)

STARTER

WEEK	DISTANCE (miles)	TIME (min)	FREQ/WK	POINTS/WK
1	1.0	18:30	5	5
2	1.0	16:30	5	5
3	1.0	15:00	5	5
4	1.5	24:30	5	7½
5	1.5	23:00	5	7½
6	1.5	22:30	5	7½

After completing the above starter program, continue with the Category I conditioning program below or, if you wish to speed up your program, take the 12-minute test of fitness. If you take the test, find your category from the table at the beginning of the chart pack (page 52). If your category is I, II, or III, continue with the appropriate category below. If your category is IV or V, follow the instructions in the note at the bottom of page 94.

CONDITIONING

FITNESS CATEGORY I   (Less than 0.80 mile on 12-minute test)

WEEK	DISTANCE (miles)	TIME (min)	FREQ/WK	POINTS/WK
7	2.0	32:00	5	10
8	2.0	31:00	5	10
9	2.5	38:30	5	12½
10	2.0	28:45	2	15½
	and			
	2.5	27:30	3	
11	2.0	28:30	3	17
	and			
	2.5	37:00	2	
12	2.5	36:00	3	21
	and			
	3.0	44:30	2	
13	2.0	28:00	2	26
	and			
	3.0	43:15	3	
14	2.5	35:00	3	27
	and			
	3.0	43:00	2	
15	3.0	43:00	5	30
16	4.0	57:00	3	33

WALKING EXERCISE PROGRAM
(age 50 and over)

CONDITIONING

FITNESS CATEGORY II   (0.80–0.99 mile on 12-minute test)

WEEK	DISTANCE (miles)	TIME (min)	FREQ/WK	POINTS/WK
7	2.5	38:30	5	12½
8	2.0	28:45	2	15½
	and			
	2.5	37:30	3	
9	2.0	28:30	3	17
	and			
	2.5	37:00	2	
10	2.0	28:00	2	26
	and			
	3.0	43:15	3	
11	2.5	35:00	3	27
	and			
	3.0	43:00	2	
12	3.0	43:00	5	30
13	4.0	57:00	3	33

FITNESS CATEGORY III   (1.0–1.24 miles on 12-minute test)

WEEK	DISTANCE (miles)	TIME (min)	FREQ/WK	POINTS/WK
7	2.5	36:00	3	21
	and			
	3.0	44:30	2	
8	2.5	35:00	3	27
	and			
	3.0	43:00	2	
9	3.0	43:00	5	30
10	4.0	57:00	3	33

After completing the progressive walking program, go to pages 107–8 and select one of the 30-point-per-week programs or develop one of your own from the point value charts beginning on page 111.

RUNNING EXERCISE PROGRAM
(age 50 and over)

STARTER *

WEEK	DISTANCE (miles)	TIME (min)	FREQ/WK	POINTS/WK
1	1.0	18:30	5	5
2	1.0	17:00	5	5
3	1.0	16:00	5	5
4	1.0	15:00	5	5
5	1.0	14:15	5	10
6	1.0	13:45	5	10

After completing the above starter program, continue with the Category I conditioning program below or, if you wish to speed up your program, take the 12-minute test of fitness. If you take the test, find your category from the table at the beginning of the chart pack (page 52). If your category is I, II, or III, continue with the appropriate category below. If your category is IV or V, follow the instructions in the note at the bottom of page 98.

* Start the program by walking, then walk and run, or run, as necessary to meet the changing time goals.

RUNNING EXERCISE PROGRAM
(age 50 and over)

CONDITIONING

FITNESS CATEGORY I   (Less than 0.80 mile on 12-minute test)

WEEK	DISTANCE (miles)	TIME (min)	FREQ/WK	POINTS/WK
7	1.5	22:00	5	15
8	1.5	20:30	5	15
9	1.5	19:30	5	15
10	1.0	11:30	1	15
	and			
	1.5	18:30	4	
11	1.0	10:45	1	21
	and			
	1.5	17:30	4	
12	1.0	10:15	1	21
	and			
	1.5	16:30	4	
13	1.5	16:00	3	27½
	and			
	2.0	22:00	2	
14	1.0	9:45	2	29
	and			
	2.0	21:15	3	
15	1.5	15:05	2	30
	and			
	2.0	20:30	3	
16	1.0	9:30	1	34
	and			
	1.5	14:25	2	
	and			
	2.0	19:55	2	

RUNNING EXERCISE PROGRAM
(age 50 and over)

CONDITIONING

FITNESS CATEGORY II   (0.80–0.99 mile on 12-minute test)

WEEK	DISTANCE (miles)	TIME (min)	FREQ/WK	POINTS/WK
7	1.5	20:30	5	15
8	1.5	19:00	5	15
9	1.0	11:30	2	16½
	and			
	1.5	17:45	3	
10	1.0	10:45	1	21
	and			
	1.5	16:45	4	
11	1.0	10:15	2	24
	and			
	1.5	22:00	3	
12	1.0	9:45	2	26
	and			
	2.0	21:00	3	
13	1.0	9:30	1	32
	and			
	1.5	14:25	2	
	and			
	2.0	19:55	2	

RUNNING EXERCISE PROGRAM
(age 50 and over)

CONDITIONING

FITNESS CATEGORY III   (1.0–1.24 miles on 12-minute test)

WEEK	DISTANCE (miles)	TIME (min)	FREQ/WK	POINTS/WK
7	1.5	19:00	5	15
8	1.0	11:30	3	18
	and			
	1.5	17:30	2	
9	1.5	15:15	3	25
	and			
	2.0	22:00	2	
10	1.0	9:30	1	32
	and			
	1.5	14:25	2	
	and			
	2.0	19:55	2	

After completing the progressive running program, go to pages 107–8 and select one of the 30-point-per-week programs or develop one of your own from the point value charts beginning on page 111.

CYCLING EXERCISE PROGRAM
(age 50 and over)

STARTER

WEEK	DISTANCE (miles)	TIME (min)	FREQ/WK	POINTS/WK
1	2.0	11:30	5	5
2	2.0	10:30	5	5
3	2.0	10:00	5	5
4	3.0	16:00	5	7½
5	3.0	15:30	5	7½
6	3.0	15:00	5	7½

After completing the above starter program, continue with the Category I conditioning program below or, if you wish to speed up your program, take the 12-minute test of fitness. If you take the test, find your category from the table at the beginning of the chart pack (page 52). If your category is I, II, or III, continue with the appropriate category below. If your category is IV or V, follow the instructions in the note at the bottom of page 100.

CONDITIONING

FITNESS CATEGORY I   (Less than 0.80 mile on 12-minute test)

WEEK	DISTANCE (miles)	TIME (min)	FREQ/WK	POINTS/WK
7	4.0	21:00	5	10
8	4.0	20:00	5	10
9	5.0	26:30	5	12½
10	5.0	25:00	1	14½
	and			
	6.0	32:00	4	
11	5.0	25:00	3	18½
	and			
	7.0	39:30	2	
12	7.0	38:00	4	22
13	5.0	24:00	2	24½
	and			
	8.0	42:00	3	
14	8.0	40:00	3	28
	and			
	10.0	57:30	1	
15	10.0	55:00	4	34
16	12.0	65:00	3	31½

CYCLING EXERCISE PROGRAM
(age 50 and over)

CONDITIONING

FITNESS CATEGORY II   (0.80–0.99 mile on 12-minute test)

WEEK	DISTANCE (miles)	TIME (min)	FREQ/WK	POINTS/WK
7	5.0	26:30	5	12½
8	5.0	25:00	1	14½
	and			
	6.0	32:00	4	
9	5.0	25:00	3	18½
	and			
	7.0	39:30	2	
10	5.0	24:00	2	24½
	and			
	8.0	42:00	3	
11	8.0	40:00	3	28
	and			
	10.0	57:30	1	
12	10.0	55:00	4	34
13	12.0	65:00	3	31½

FITNESS CATEGORY III   (1.0–1.24 miles on 12-minute test)

WEEK	DISTANCE (miles)	TIME (min)	FREQ/WK	POINTS/WK
7	7.0	38:00	4	22
8	8.0	40:00	3	28
	and			
	10.0	57:30	1	
9	10.0	55:00	4	34
10	12.0	65:00	3	31½

After completing the progressive cycling program, go to pages 107–8 and select one of the 30-point-per-week programs or develop one of your own from the point value charts beginning on page 111.

SWIMMING EXERCISE PROGRAM
(age 50 and over)

Overhand Crawl *

STARTER

WEEK	DISTANCE (yards)	TIME (min)	FREQ/WK	POINTS/WK
1	100	2:30	5	4
2	150	3:45	5	5
3	175	4:15	5	6
4	200	4:45	5	7½
5	200	4:30	5	7½
6	200	4:15	5	7½

After completing the above starter program, continue with the Category I conditioning program below or, if you wish to speed up your program, take the 12-minute test of fitness. If you take the test, find your category from the table at the beginning of the chart pack (page 52). If your category is I, II, or III, continue with the appropriate category below. If your category is IV or V, follow the instructions in the note at the bottom of page 102.

* Breaststroke is less demanding and so is backstroke. Butterfly is considerably more demanding.

CONDITIONING

Fitness Category I   (Less than 0.80 mile on 12-minute test)

WEEK	DISTANCE (yards)	TIME (min)	FREQ/WK	POINTS/WK
7	200	5:45	5	10
8	250	5:30	5	10
9	300	7:15	5	12½
10	300	6:45	5	12½
11	400	9:45	5	17½
12	400	9:30	2	19
	and			
	500	12:00	3	
13	400	9:15	2	22
	and			
	600	13:45	3	
14	500	11:30	2	26
	and			
	700	16:30	3	
15	700	16:00	5	30
16	800	18:00	4	30

SWIMMING EXERCISE PROGRAM
(age 50 and over)

Overhand Crawl *

CONDITIONING

FITNESS CATEGORY II   (0.80–0.99 mile on 12-minute test)

WEEK	DISTANCE (yards)	TIME (min)	FREQ/WK	POINTS/WK
7	300	7:15	5	12½
8	300	6:45	5	12½
9	400	9:45	5	17½
10	400	9:15	2	22
	and			
	600	13:45	3	
11	500	11:30	2	26
	and			
	700	16:30	3	
12	700	16:00	5	30
13	800	18:00	4	30

FITNESS CATEGORY III   (1.0–1.24 miles on 12-minute test)

WEEK	DISTANCE (yards)	TIME (min)	FREQ/WK	POINTS/WK
7	400	9:30	2	19
	and			
	500	12:30	3	
8	500	11:30	2	26
	and			
	700	16:30	3	
9	700	16:00	5	30
10	800	18:00	4	30

* Breaststroke is less demanding and so is backstroke. Butterfly is considerably more demanding.

After completing the progressive swimming program, go to pages 107–8 and select one of the 30-point-per-week programs or develop one of your own from the point value charts beginning on page 111.

STATIONARY RUNNING EXERCISE PROGRAM
(age 50 and over)

STARTER

WEEK	DURATION (min)	STEPS/MIN *	FREQ/WK	POINTS/WK
1	1:30	70–80	5	—
2	2:30	70–80	5	4
3	2:30	70–80	5	4
4	5:00	70–80	5	7½
5	5:00	70–80	5	7½
6	5:00	70–80	5	7½

After completing the above starter program, continue with the Category I conditioning program below or, if you wish to speed up your program, take the 12-minute test of fitness. If you take the test, find your category from the table at the beginning of the chart pack (page 52). If your category is I, II, or III, continue with the appropriate category below. If your category is IV or V, follow the instructions in the note at the bottom of page 104.

* Count only when the left foot hits the floor. Feet must be brought at least eight inches from the floor.

CONDITIONING

FITNESS CATEGORY I   (Less than 0.80 mile on 12-minute test)

WEEK	DURATION (min)	STEPS/MIN *	FREQ/WK	POINTS/WK
7	7:30	70–80	5	11¼
8	7:30	70–80	5	11¼
9	10:00	70–80	5	15
10	10:00	70–80	5	15
11	10:00	70–80	5	15
12	12:30	70–80	5	18¾
13	10:00 (1x in A.M.) and	70–80	2	23¼
	10:00 (1x in P.M.) and	70–80		
	12:30	70–80	3	
14	10:00 (1x in A.M.) and	70–80	2	25½
	10:00 (1x in P.M.) and	70–80		
	15:00	70–80	3	
15	12:30 (1x in A.M.) and	70–80	2	28½
	12:30 (1x in P.M.) and	70–80		
	15:00	70–80	3	
16	20:00	70–80	4	32

* Count only when the left foot hits the floor. Feet must be brought at least eight inches from the floor.

STATIONARY RUNNING EXERCISE PROGRAM
(age 50 and over)

CONDITIONING

FITNESS CATEGORY II   (0.80–0.99 mile on 12-minute test)

WEEK	DURATION (min)	STEPS/MIN *	FREQ/WK	POINTS/WK
7	10:00	70–80	5	15
8	10:00	70–80	5	15
9	10:00	70–80	5	15
10	10:00 (1x in A.M.) and	70–80	2	23¼
	10:00 (1x in P.M.) and	70–80		
	12:30	70–80	3	
11	10:00 (1x in A.M.) and	70–80	2	25½
	10:00 (1x in P.M.) and	70–80		
	15:00	70–80	3	
12	12:30 (1x in A.M.) and	70–80	2	28½
	12:30 (1x in P.M.) and	70–80		
	15:00	70–80	3	
13	20:00	70–80	4	32

* Count only when the left foot hits the floor. Feet must be brought at least eight inches from the floor.

FITNESS CATEGORY III   (1.0–1.24 miles on 12-minute test)

WEEK	DURATION (min)	STEPS/MIN *	FREQ/WK	POINTS/WK
7	12:30	70–80	5	18¾
8	10:00 (1x in A.M.) and	70–80	2	25½
	10:00 (1x in P.M.) and	70–80		
	15:00	70–80	3	
9	12:30 (1x in A.M.) and	70–80	2	28½
	12:30 (1x in P.M.) and	70–80		
	15:00	70–80	3	
10	20:00	70–80	4	32

* Count only when the left foot hits the floor. Feet must be brought at least eight inches from the floor.

After completing the progressive stationary running program, go to pages 107–8 and select one of the 30-point-per-week programs or develop one of your own from the point value charts beginning on page 111.

HANDBALL/BASKETBALL/SQUASH EXERCISE PROGRAM
(age 50 and over)

STARTER

WEEK	TIME (min) *	FREQ/WK	POINTS/WK
1	7:30	5	5
2	7:30	5	5
3	10:00	5	7½
4	10:00	5	7½
5	12:30	5	10
6	12:30	5	10

After completing the above starter program, continue with the Category I conditioning program below or, if you wish to speed up your program, take the 12-minute test of fitness. If you take the test, find your category from the table at the beginning of the chart pack (page 52). If your category is I, II, or III, continue with the appropriate category below. If your category is IV or V, follow the instructions in the note at the bottom of page 106.

* Continuous exercise. Do not count breaks, time-outs, etc.

CONDITIONING

FITNESS CATEGORY I   (Less than 0.80 mile on 12-minute test)

WEEK	TIME (min) *	FREQ/WK	POINTS/WK
7	15:00	5	11¼
8	15:00	5	11¼
9	20:00	5	15
10	20:00	5	15
11	25:00	5	18¾
12	25:00	5	18¾
13	20:00 and 30:00	1 4	21
14	20:00 and 30:00	1 4	24
15	35:00 and 40:00	3 2	27¾
16	40:00	5	30

* Continuous exercise. Do not count breaks, time-outs, etc.

HANDBALL/BASKETBALL/SQUASH EXERCISE PROGRAM
(age 50 and over)

CONDITIONING

FITNESS CATEGORY II   (0.80–0.99 mile on 12-minute test)

WEEK	TIME (min) *	FREQ/WK	POINTS/WK
7	20:00	5	15
8	20:00	5	15
9	25:00	5	18¾
10	20:00 and	1	21
	30:00	4	
11	20:00 and	1	
	30:00	4	24
12	35:00 and	3	27¾
	40:00	2	
13	40:00	5	30

* Continuous exercise. Do not count breaks, time-outs, etc.

FITNESS CATEGORY III   (1.0–1.24 miles on 12-minute test)

WEEK	TIME (min) *	FREQ/WK	POINTS/WK
7	25:00	5	18¾
8	20:00 and	1	24
	30:00	4	
9	35:00 and	3	27¾
	40:00	2	
10	40:00	5	30

* Continuous exercise. Do not count breaks, time-outs, etc.

After completing the progressive handball/basketball/squash program, go to pages 107–8 and select one of the 30-point-per-week programs or develop one of your own from the point value charts beginning on page 111.

PROGRAMS FOR CATEGORIES IV AND V
(all ages)

FITNESS LEVEL IS SATISFACTORY AT THE OUTSET. THE ONLY REQUIREMENT IS TO MAINTAIN FITNESS USING ONE OF THE FOLLOWING EXERCISE PROGRAMS.

	DISTANCE (miles)	TIME (min) REQUIREMENT	FREQ/WK	POINTS/WK
WALKING	2.0	24:00–29:00	8	32
	or			
	3.0	36:00–43:30	5	30
	or			
	4.0	58:00–79:59	5	35
	or			
	4.0	48:00–58:00	3	33
RUNNING	1.0	6:30– 7:59	6	30
	or			
	1.5	12:00–14:59	5	30
	or			
	1.5	9:45–11:59	4	30
	or			
	2.0	16:00–19:59	4	36
	or			
	2.0	13:00–15:59	3	33
CYCLING	5.0	15:00–19:59	6	30
	or			
	6.0	18:00–23:59	5	30
	or			
	7.0	21:00–27:59	4	36
	or			
	8.0	24:00–31:59	3	31
	YARDS			
SWIMMING	500	8:20–12:59	8	32
	or			
	600	10:00–14:59	6	30
	or			
	800	13:20–19:59	4	30
	or			
	1000	16:40–24:59	3	31½

PROGRAMS FOR CATEGORIES IV AND V
(all ages)

	DURATION (min)	STEPS/MIN *	FREQ/WK	POINTS/WK
STATIONARY RUNNING	10:00 in A.M. and	70–80	5	30
	10:00 in P.M. or	70–80		
	15:00 or	70–80	7	30
	15:00 or	80–90	5	30
	20:00	70–80	4	32

* Count only when the left foot hits the floor. Feet must be brought at least eight inches from the floor.

HANDBALL BASKETBALL SQUASH	40:00 or	—	5	30
	50:00 or	—	4	30
	70:00	—	3	30

SUGGESTED PROGRESSIVE WALKING PROGRAM FOR CARDIAC PATIENTS—A

(Minimal Disease—Uncomplicated)

WEEKS	DISTANCE (miles)	TIME GOAL (min)	FREQ/WK	POINTS/WK
1–2	1.0	20:00	5	—
3–4	1.0	17:30	5	5
5–6	1.0	15:00	5	5
7–8	1.5	23:00	5	7½
9–10	1.5	22:30	5	7½
11–12	2.0	31.00	5	10
13–14	2.0	30:00	5	10
15–16	1.5	21:30	5	15
17–18	1.5	21:00	5	15
19–20	2.0	28:45	3	22
	and			
	2.5	36:00	2	
21–22	2.0	28:30	3	22
	and			
	2.5	35:45	2	
23–24	2.5	35:30	4	26
	and			
	3.0	43:15	1	
25–26	2.5	35:15	3	27
	and			
	3.0	43:15	2	
27–28	2.5	35:00	3	27
	and			
	3.0	42:30	2	
29–30	3.0	42:00	5	30
31–32	4.0	55:00	3	33

MINIMAL REQUIREMENTS TO MAINTAIN FITNESS AFTER
COMPLETION OF CONDITIONING PROGRAM—A

DISTANCE (miles)	TIME GOAL (min)	FREQ/WK	POINTS/WK
1.5 (twice a day)	18:00–21:44	5	30
or 2.0	24:00–28:59	8	32
or 3.0	36:00–43:29	5	30
or 4.0	48:00–57:59	3	33
or 5.0	72:30–99:59	4	36

SUGGESTED PROGRESSIVE WALKING PROGRAM FOR CARDIAC PATIENTS—B

(Moderate Disease)

WEEKS	DISTANCE (miles)	TIME GOAL (min)	FREQ/WK	POINTS/WK
1–2	1.0	24:00	5	—
3–4	1.0	20:00	5	—
5–6	1.0	18:00	5	5
7–8	1.0	16:00	5	5
9–10	1.5	25:00	5	7½
11–12	1.5	24:00	5	7½
13–14	2.0	33:00	5	10
15–16	2.0	32:00	5	10
17–18	1.5	23:00	2	10½
	and			
	2.5	40:00	3	
19–20	1.5	22:30	2	12
	and			
	3.0	47:00	3	
21–22	2.5	38:00	2	15½
	and			
	3.5	54:00	3	
23–24	2.5	36:00	3	21
	and			
	3.0	44:00	2	
25–26	3.0	43:15	3	26
	and			
	4.0	61:00	2	
27–28	3.0	43:15	3	26
	and			
	4.0	60:00	2	
29–30	3.0	43:00	5	30
31–32	4.0	57:45	3	33

MINIMUM REQUIREMENTS TO MAINTAIN FITNESS AFTER COMPLETION OF CONDITIONING PROGRAM—B

DISTANCE (miles)	TIME GOAL (min)	FREQ/WK	POINTS/WK
1.5 (twice a day)	18:00–21:44	5	30
or 2.0	24:00–28:59	8	32
or 3.0	36:00–43:29	5	30
or 4.0	48:00–57:59	3	33
or 4.0	58:00–79:59	4	28
or 5.0	72:30–99:59	3	27

POINT VALUE CHARTS

For a more complete breakdown of these point values, see Appendix.

WALKING

1 Mile	POINTS
19:59—14:30 min	1
14:29—12:00 min	2

1.5 Miles	POINTS
29:59—21:45 min	1½
21:44—18:00 min	3

2 Miles	POINTS
40:00 min or longer	1*
39:59—29:00 min	2
28:59—24:00 min	4

2.5 Miles	POINTS
50:00 min or longer	1*
49:59—36:15 min	2½
36:14—30:00 min	5

3 Miles	POINTS
60:00 min or longer	1½*
59:59—43:30 min	3
43:29—36:00 min	6

3.5 Miles	POINTS
70:00 min or longer	1½*
69:59—50:45 min	3½
50:44—42:00 min	7

4 Miles	POINTS
80:00 min or longer	4*
79:59—58:00 min	7
57:59—48:00 min	11

4.5 Miles	POINTS
90 min or longer	4½*
89:59—65:15 min	8
65:14—54:00 min	12½

5 Miles	POINTS
100:00 min or longer	5*
99:59—72:30 min	9
72:29—60:00 min	14

RUNNING

1 Mile	POINTS
14:29—12:00 min	2
11:59—10:00 min	3
9:59— 8:00 min	4
7:59— 6:30 min	5
under 6:30 min	6

2 Miles	POINTS
28:59—24:00 min	4
23:59—20:00 min	7
19:59—16:00 min	9
15:59—13:00 min	11
under 13:00 min	13

1.5 Miles	POINTS
21:44—18:00 min	3
17:59—15:00 min	4½
14:59—12:00 min	6
11:59— 9:45 min	7½
under 9:45 min	9

2.5 Miles	POINTS
36:14—30:00 min	5
29:59—25:00 min	9
24:59—20:00 min	11½
19:59—16:15 min	14
under 16:15 min	16½

* Exercise of sufficient duration to be of cardiovascular benefit. At this speed, ordinarily no training effect would occur. However, the duration is of such extent that a training effect does begin to occur.

POINT VALUE CHARTS

For a more complete breakdown of these point values, see Appendix.

RUNNING (CONTINUED)

3 Miles	POINTS	4 Miles	POINTS
43:29—36:00 min	6	57:59—48:00 min	11
35:59—30:00 min	11	47.59—40:00 min	15
29:59—24:00 min	14	39:59—32:00 min	19
23:59—19:30 min	17	31:59—26:00 min	23
under 19:30 min	20	under 26:00 min	27

3.5 Miles	POINTS	5 Miles	POINTS
50:44—42:00 min	7	72:29—60:00 min	10
41:59—35:00 min	13	59:59—50:00 min	15
34:59—28:00 min	16½	49:59—40:00 min	20
27:59—22:45 min	20	39:59—32:30 min	25
under 22:45 min	23½	under 32:30 min	30

CYCLING

2 Miles	POINTS	6 Miles	POINTS
12 min or longer	0	36 min or longer	1*
11:59—8:00 min	1	35:59—24:00 min	3
7:59— 6:00 min	2	23:59—18:00 min	6
under 6:00 min	3	under 18:00 min	9

3 Miles	POINTS	8 Miles	POINTS
18 min or longer	0	48 min or longer	3½*
17:59—12:00 min	1½	47:59—32:00 min	6½
11:59— 9:00 min	3	31:59—24:00 min	10½
under 9:00 min	4½	under 24:00 min	14½

4 Miles	POINTS	10 Miles	POINTS
24 min or longer	0	60 min or longer	5½*
23:59—16:00 min	2	59:59—40:00 min	8½
15:59—12:00 min	4	39:59—30:00 min	13½
under 12:00 min	6	under 30:00 min	18½

5 Miles	POINTS
30 min or longer	1*
29:59—20:00 min	2½
19:59—15:00 min	5
under 15:00 min	7½

* Exercise of sufficient duration to be of cardiovascular benefit. At this speed, ordinarily no training effect would occur. However, the duration is of such extent that a training effect does begin to occur.

POINT VALUE CHARTS

For a more complete breakdown of these point values, see Appendix.

SWIMMING

200 Yards	POINTS	600 Yards	POINTS
6:40 min or longer	0	20:00 min or longer	1½*
6:39— 5:00 min	1	19:59—15:00 min	4
4:59— 3:20 min	1½	14:59—10:00 min	5
under 3:20 min	2½	under 10:00 min	7½

300 Yards	POINTS	700 Yards	POINTS
10:00 min or longer	1*	23:20 min or longer	1½*
9:59— 7:30 min	1½	23:19—17:30 min	4½
7:29— 5:00 min	2½	17:29—11:40 min	6
under 5:00 min	3½	under 11:40 min	8½

400 Yards	POINTS	800 Yards	POINTS
13:20 min or longer	1*	26:40 min or longer	2¼*
13:19—10:00 min	2½	26:39—20:00 min	5¾
9:59— 6:40 min	3½	19:59—13:20 min	7¼
under 6:40 min	5	under 13:20 min	10¾

500 Yards	POINTS	1000 Yards	POINTS
16:40 min or longer	1*	33:20 min or longer	4*
16:39—12:30 min	3	33:19—25:00 min	8¼
12:29— 8:20 min	4	24:59—16:40 min	10½
under 8:20 min	6	under 16:40 min	14½

* Exercise of sufficient duration to be of cardiovascular benefit. At this speed, ordinarily no training effect would occur. However, the duration is of such extent that a training effect does begin to occur.

POINT VALUE CHARTS

For a more complete breakdown of these point values, see Appendix.

HANDBALL/BASKETBALL/SQUASH *

DURATION	POINTS		DURATION	POINTS
10	1½		55	8¼
15	2¼		60	9
20	3		65	9¾
25	3¾		70	10½
30	4½		75	11¼
35	5¼		80	12
40	6		85	12¾
45	6¾		90	13½
50	7½			

* Continuous exercise. Do not include breaks, time-outs, etc.

STATIONARY RUNNING

TIME	*60-70 STEPS/MIN	POINTS	*70-80 STEPS/MIN	POINTS	*80-90 STEPS/MIN	POINTS
2:30			175-200	¾	200-225	1
5:00	300-350	1¼	350-400	1½	400-450	2
7:30			525-600	2¼	600-675	3
10:00	600-700	2½	700-800	3	800-900	4
12:30			785-1000	3¾	1000-1125	5
15:00	900-1050	3¾	1050-1200	4½	1200-1350	6
17:30			1225-1400	6¾	1400-1575	8½
20:00	1200-1400	7	1400-1600	8	1600-1800	10

* Count only when the left foot hits the floor. Feet must be brought at least eight inches from the floor.

7: Tips and Safeguards

THAT PROVERBIAL OUNCE of prevention also applies to aerobics. This chapter is basically a discussion of possible problems occurring with an exercise program, along with tips on how to avoid them—and hints on how to treat them if they occur.

FOOT TROUBLE

Since foot and ankle troubles are the most frequently encountered exercise problems, they deserve special attention.

The human foot is a marvel of engineering, but it is not well adapted for pounding hard pavements or hard floors. Because of this, some runners develop back pains, leg muscle pains, and swollen ankles. Others develop Achilles tendonitis—soreness and inflammation of the big tendon connecting the heel with the calf. Tendonitis even strikes well-trained athletes, usually without warning, and it may take several weeks to clear up.

To prevent some of these problems, it helps to have a proper warm-up, as discussed in Chapter Five. Occasionally tendonitis occurs when a runner resumes regular workouts after a long layoff. In such cases, it is just as important to stress progressive reentry into the exercise program as it is a proper warm-up.

Stationary running is harder on the feet and ankles than normal running, particularly when it is done in bare feet. Without the support provided by the heel of the shoe, you become a prime candidate for tendonitis and other ankle problems. So keep your shoes on for indoor running.

The so-called "jogger's heel" also occurs occasionally in adult runners. The symptom is a very sore heel caused by landing hard on the heel while running on a concrete or solid surface. To avoid this problem: 1) run flatfooted, touching down with more of the entire sole; 2) avoid running on hard surfaces; and 3) use a cushion-soled shoe.

A more troublesome, but fortunately rare complication is the stress or march fracture of the foot. This happens mostly to older people, whose bones are more brittle. But it may occur at any age.

The sign of a stress or march fracture is a sharp and persistent pain in the foot. It is not a serious matter and with immobilization it usually heals within weeks. Nonetheless, it should be x-rayed, properly treated, and complete healing should be confirmed by your doctor before you resume exercise.

Anytime you develop a problem with your feet and ankles, the best immediate treatment is to reduce the speed and duration of your exercise. If this doesn't work, stop exercising completely and rest the affected part. (Many people follow this rule: If exercise aggravates the pain, stop; if the pain disappears with exercise, continue.)

If your problems persist, it may be necessary to change to another exercise program. For example, a middle-aged man from Houston writes:

Even though I responded well to the running program and was able to meet all the time requirements, my arthritic ankles couldn't stand the strain. My physician said I had to stop running. With his consent I started cycling and can now cycle five miles in less than 20:00 minutes—and the pain in my ankles completely disappeared.

The proper running style is also of great help in avoiding foot and leg problems. In general, people run too much on either their heels or their toes. I encourage people to run mostly flatfooted.

After the flatfooted touchdown, roll the weight forward on the foot, from heel to toe. Don't run with rigid knees and allow the slightly flexed knee to absorb some of the impact when the foot strikes the ground. Avoid bouncing when running. You can determine how much you are bouncing by watching a stationary object. Let the arms swing comfortably at your side, parallel to your body movement.

Another important point, as I've mentioned before, is the running surface. For stationary running I would recommend a soft rug, preferably with a spongy underlayer. For outdoor running, unfortunately, you have to use whatever is available. A dirt road is good; a quarter mile track is better (particularly if it is covered with the new, resilient, Olympic-type plastic surface) but the best surface is a smooth, well-kept grass field. Since the ideal surface is rarely available, the necessity for good, cushioned-sole shoes is re-emphasized.

Picking the right kind of running shoes is probably the biggest factor in avoiding ankle, foot and leg problems. Light, crosscountry shoes are good for running on hard surfaces, but I prefer special long-distance, ripple-sole shoes. The best of these have cushioned innersoles made of some spongy material that gives springy resilience to your step. Avoid standard basketball or tennis shoes, which have an unusually hard sole.

As for socks, it's entirely up to you whether you prefer cotton or nylon. One drawback of nylon socks is that they do not absorb perspiration. Cotton absorbs perspiration, but does not insulate as well against friction.

If your shoes fit well, you may not even need socks. In long-distance running, socks mean extra weight, and some athletes—particularly marathon runners—prefer to run without them. There are insoles that can be inserted in your shoes to reduce friction and blisters.

In case blisters do occur, treat them immediately after running. Keep your feet clean and dry, and the toenails closely clipped.

With these guidelines, you stand an excellent chance of minimizing foot and ankle problems.

KNEE AND LEG PROBLEMS

The most common leg problem with runners is "shin splints." The symptoms are pain and tightness in the muscles in the front of the leg below the knee. Shin splints usually result from running on hard surfaces with hard shoes and are successfully treated by the reverse, that is soft surfaces and cushioned-sole shoes.

Knee problems commonly occur in conditioning programs, particularly among people with old knee injuries. However, even with severe knee and joint problems, some people have been able to run effectively. Let me give you an example.

Sergeant Elmer Jones, a 51-year-old retired member of the USAF has been running with us for over 1½ years. Several years ago, he had an operation on his left knee to correct some chronic changes occurring in the joint. The left kneecap and some cartilage had to be removed. However, progressive exercise strengthened and stabilized his knee and just a few weeks ago he ran 1½ miles in 10:28 minutes—placing him in the Excellent fitness category.

Running distances exceeding one mile on small, unbanked tracks, requiring 25 or more laps to the mile, often causes pain in ankles and knees. For this reason it is preferable to do your outdoor running on larger tracks or on indoor tracks with banked curves. If no such track is available, you can minimize the problems of the smaller track by running 25 laps in one direction and then reversing your direction if you desire to run further. Remember also that a good pair of shoes is just as important for the protection of the knees as it is for the protection of the ankles when you must exercise on a hard surface.

Muscle cramps or spasms in the legs are not uncommon during the early stages of a conditioning program. A muscle only partially conditioned is especially likely to develop cramps. However, this is a transient problem, usually disappearing as a good state of fitness is reached.

BACK TROUBLE

A few individuals who limited their exercise program exclusively to jogging on hard surfaces have written complaining of pain in the lower region of the back. This is not a serious matter, but such discomfort can usually be avoided by supplementing jogging with some calisthenic exercise, notably 15–20 repetitions of both sit-ups with the knees bent and push-ups. These exercises strengthen the back and help to relieve back pain. Cyclists also complain of back aches, and I recommend that they try the same calisthenic routines.

SWIMMERS' PROBLEMS

Swimmers sometimes suffer from a chronic infection of the ear canal. This used to be a common complaint before the chlorination of swimming pools became general practice. If it does occur, see your doctor and have the infection treated. If you find that you are frequently troubled with such infections, swab out your ears after each swim with cotton (or a cotton swab) dipped in alcohol.

Some swimmers develop chronic sinus trouble. An effective precaution is the use of a nose clip while swimming. Competition swimmers report that this increases breathing resistance and tends to lower their performance. But the difference is so slight that I recommend using the nose clip for non-competitive swimming, particularly if the swimming is done as part of an aerobic conditioning program.

EXCESS FATIGUE

A man from Ohio wrote: "Your aerobics program is really great! I run a mile five days a week and now I can go home, go to bed at 6:30, and sleep the rest of the night."

He obviously had missed the point.

Being pleasantly tired for a short period after exercise is one thing. You'd normally expect that. But feeling worn out all the time is something else. Chronic fatigue is a sign that you are exercising at a pace for which you are not yet ready. It is a sign that you need some rest.

I advised my Ohio correspondent to ease up on his exercise until he could get by with seven or eight hours of sleep. "Drop back a couple of weeks in the chart or stay at a level you can tolerate without feeling tired all the time," I wrote him. "Aerobics shouldn't make you constantly sleepy; it should help keep you awake."

Aerobics can be a highly effective cure for ordinary types of insomnia. But the idea is to make you sleep better—not longer. Because exercise reduces your tensions, it helps you to sleep more easily and more deeply. It increases the efficiency of your sleep, so you feel more rested on less sleep. Combined with the general invigoration of your whole system, this should give you extra alertness during your waking hours.

If you do feel overly tired during the later weeks of your conditioning program, you can probably lick the problem by changing your schedule. For example, schedule one resting day after two days of exercise. Of course, to maintain a high level of fitness you should exercise at least four times per week. But that doesn't mean four consecutive days.

There's another way to lick fatigue problems and still earn enough points.

The speed of exercise (the intensity of your workout) may contribute more to fatigue than the duration. So if you have a persistent fatigue problem, I suggest that you exercise at a slower rate for a longer time. You still earn your points but with less strain.

For example, I like to run three miles during the lunch hour several days a week. My time is usually 20:00–21:00 minutes. This is worth 15 points. However, if it is really hot, as at times it can be in south Texas, I tend to get overly fatigued and may be tired the remainder of the day. By running the same distance but slowing the time to 23:30–23:59 minutes, I don't become fatigued at all. In fact, I sometimes feel guilty and feel as though I didn't work out hard enough. But I still get 15 points and I'm wide awake the rest of the day.

Another personal example: At times I have to miss my noon workout due to a multitude of commitments, and I may end up mentally exhausted before 5:00 P.M. Yet, I have several hours of work to accomplish that evening. If I run 1½–2 miles prior to dinner, shower and clean up, it completely revitalizes me. It may be purely psychosomatic but try it, it works!

One of my correspondents summed up all the problems, difficulties and benefits of aerobics this way: "After eight weeks on the conditioning program, I feel younger, stronger, and more alive. And my problems—the ones that looked so big before—well, they haven't gone away. But somehow they look smaller."

Of course, these are subjective reactions. But they also reflect real changes: the strengthening of the heart and lungs, improved circulation, and the ability to distribute more oxygen throughout the body—all the changes that really count.

8: Aerobic Therapy

To MAINTAIN A satisfactory level of fitness and show improvement in various medical conditions, you should average a minimum of 30 points per week.

"And what's so wonderful about 30 points? Why do you set this figure as a goal?"

Let me try to answer this often-asked question. Thirty points per week is enough of a demand on the body to make it respond. With 30 points your body will show definite signs of conditioning—you will fatigue less easily, your heart and lungs will work more efficiently, your capacity for transporting oxygen will increase, and you will probably look and feel better.

Many people who faithfully earn their 30 points each week think of it as a type of health insurance. In a way it is. It will enable you to live a healthier and more productive life, but it is not the fountain of youth. It will help you to lose weight, but you won't lose it rapidly unless you diet along with your exercise program. It will decrease the severity and frequency of many of your medical problems although it may not eliminate them altogether. And as I have already mentioned, it is no guarantee against heart disease, but it is of value in the prevention and rehabilitation of this disease. In that sense, maintaining your 30-point-per-week exercise routine is buying you a lot of health insurance.

Now let us consider the use of aerobic conditioning in treating selected medical problems.

HEART AND BLOOD VESSEL DISEASE

At least one million Americans die each year from heart and blood vessel disorders—600,000, which adds up to one death every 50 seconds, from coronary disease alone. Coronary heart disease has a number of causes: heredity, stress, diet, smoking and inactivity. Some of these causes cannot be changed but patterns of inactivity definitely can be changed. Fortunately, more and more people are starting exercise programs as a means of practicing both preventive and rehabilitative medicine.

In the practice of rehabilitative medicine, physicians are beginning to encourage progressive exercise for selected patients with heart disease.

For example, Master Sergeant J. D. Mott, USAF, suffered a severe heart attack at the age of 41. At that time he was overweight, anxious, smoking heavily and inactive. He survived his heart attack, and four months later decided to join the aerobics program we were conducting for cardiac patients. At that point, his only symptom was occasional chest pain.

Sergeant Mott was placed into the walking program for cardiac patients, moderate disease. In addition, he was placed on a low-cholesterol diet and was encouraged to give up smoking.

His exercise program consisted exclusively of walking, progressing from one to four miles daily. After 12 months, all of his symptoms had disappeared, and the electrocardiogram was normal except for evidence of the old heart attack. At that time, Sergeant Mott was able to switch from the cardiac rehabilitation program to the regular aerobic conditioning program, and he started running. "Never felt better," he said, as he worked happily toward his 30–50-point-per-week goal.

After two years of such conditioning, an x-ray study of his heart showed that he had developed unusually good "collateral" circulation in his coronary system. His working capacity also had increased, and the progress of his potentially crippling and even fatal disease had apparently been slowed.

Another remarkable recovery was made by my neighbor, Mr. Bill Linder. About two years ago, Bill and I were taking an afternoon walk. Whenever we came to a hill, I noticed that Bill would grab his left elbow and complain of pain.

"Oh, it's just that old arthritis," he explained.

But I noticed that the "arthritis" bothered him only on the uphill parts of the walk. That seemed odd indeed. I began to suspect that, since the pain occurred only under stress, it might be "referred" pain from a heart condition. This type of pain, can occur almost anywhere in the upper part of the body.

I suggested to Bill that he have an exercise electrocardiogram.

He just laughed. For years he thought that his pain was arthritis. His electrocardiogram had always been normal.

"Did anyone ever check your electrocardiogram while you were exercising?" I asked.

No, Bill admitted. His doctor had only tested him in a resting condition. I promptly made arrangements for him to have an exercise electrocardiogram—the so-called Masters two-step Test. Under stress, the ECG showed clear signs of moderate to severe heart disease.

Unfortunately, such tests are not normally given with routine checkups. Perhaps we need a revamping of standard procedures or the establishment of special cardiac diagnostic centers to look for "hidden" heart disease. If I had not, by sheer chance, noticed Bill's elbow-grabbing on the uphill stretch, his condition might have remain undetected and untreated. One day he simply might have collapsed with a serious and perhaps fatal attack. Of course, everyone would have said that there had been no previous warning.

Under the supervision of his doctor, Bill started a mild, progressive walking program. After ten months, the progress of his disease had been altered and symptomatically he had improved. His ECG had reverted to normal—even with exercise. Apparently, aerobic exercise had sufficiently improved the blood supply to his heart to change the natural course of his disease.

It goes without saying that the early rehabilitative exercise programs for cardiac patients must remain quite mild. If the patient drives too hard, he may push himself to a point his damaged heart is unable to tolerate. For this reason, it is advisable to recommend to heart patients that they exercise at a level which does not cause their heart rate to exceed the age-adjusted rates listed below. This is particularly important during the early stages of a cardiac rehabilitation program.

MAXIMAL HEART RATES IN CARDIAC REHABILITATION PROGRAMS

Age (Years)	Heart Rate (Beats Per Minute)
Under 30	150
30–34	145
35–39	140
40–44	135
45–49	135
50–54	130
55–59	125
60–64	120
65+	120

A crude way to estimate the maximal heart rate during exercise is to take the pulse during the first ten seconds after exercise and multiply that number by six. However, more sophisticated monitoring methods are available today. One is an electronic device worn by the patient during exercise which sounds a warning through an earphone when his heart rate exceeds a preset limit. Soon to be available is a stationary bicycle with a built-in monitor. As the patient grabs the handlebar, he closes a circuit and can read his heart rate continuously on a meter.

Another important contributory factor to the development of coronary heart disease is a high blood-cholesterol level. The usual way to combat this condition is through diets low in cholesterol and animal fats.

However, several studies have recently shown that exercise, too, may play a role. This lowering effect may be seen in subjects involved in endurance activities even though their diets remain unchanged. To the contrary, exercise programs that tend to build large muscle mass may cause an increase in blood cholesterol levels.

Many patients with high blood pressure have responded well to aerobic therapy. Among my patients at Wilford Hall, I'd like to single out 45-year-old Lieutenant Colonel Gregory Skafidas. Two years ago he joined our program and at that time he had a blood pressure of 180/118. Over the next year, he lost 30 pounds on the aerobics program and his blood pressure dropped to 132/80. He then entered our city-wide ten-mile marathon, finishing in 72 minutes.

Now, two years later, Colonel Skafidas is averaging over 100 points per week and is a living example of the benefits of aerobic therapy.

A mechanism similar to that which restores coronary circulation in damaged hearts also operates in blood vessels in the body. The legs, for example, are frequently affected by blood vessel obstructions, and such conditions can in some instances be helped by exercise.

It should be noted, however, that not all cases of blood vessel disease respond to aerobics. For example, some sufferers from varicose veins claim that exercise aggravated their condition. Others have clearly benefited. Caution and close supervision are therefore advised in using exercise therapy in patients with blood vessel disease.

A moderately successful case of aerobic therapy for advanced vascular disease involved one of our 38-year-old patients with intermittent claudication, a blood vessel ailment causing pain in the legs with even minimal exertion. When he was first studied in our laboratory, he was unable to walk more than a few yards without severe leg pain. In fact, he had difficulty supporting his own weight for more than three minutes without intolerable pain.

He was placed into a very slow walking program and gradually, over a period of many months, his persistence paid off. The effort of walking forced an improvement in the blood supply to his legs. Slowly this new collateral circulation was able to take over, at least partly, the function of the damaged vessels. At the end of his therapy, he was able to walk a distance of one mile without incapacitating pain.

For blood vessel disease, too, I should like to stress the preventive role of aerobics. Prime candidates for blood vessel problems are people who spend a lot of time on their feet without vigorous movement, thereby placing a stress on the blood vessels in their legs. Salesmen standing long hours behind the counter, dentists bending over their patients all day, traffic cops restricted to an intersection—these are the kind of occupations with built-in risk of blood vessel disease.

LUNG DISEASE

Because aerobic exercise improves the efficiency of breathing, it is of value in treating some patients with pulmonary emphysema.

This ailment, frequently related to smoking, is now reaching epidemic proportions in the United States. Since it progressively deprives the patient of lung capacity it is important for him to adequately utilize whatever lung capacity he has remaining. Aerobics helps to accomplish this by increasing the ability to move air in and out of the lungs, by improving oxygen distribution throughout the body, and by providing for more efficient oxygen extraction in the tissues.

At Wilford Hall Hospital we have seen several emphysema patients who had been almost completely incapacitated by their disease restored to a level of competence which enabled them to lead productive lives. One of these patients is now able to walk a mile in 16 minutes.

MISCELLANEOUS MEDICAL PROBLEMS

The broad applicability of exercise therapy, and of aerobics in particular, rests on the fact that such exercise affects the total organism by improving the circulation and oxygen supply to both diseased and normal tissues, by increasing muscle tone and strength, and by decreasing body fat deposits.

In diabetes, for example, the reduction of fat through exercise apparently is a change which improves the body's ability to handle sugar. As a result, some diabetic patients (particularly those with adult onset diabetes) have been able to reduce their insulin requirement after starting a regular exercise program.

I have repeatedly pointed to the fact that exercise is a natural relaxant. This alone is highly beneficial in many clinical conditions. Ulcer patients, for example, probably owe their improvement to the fact they become less tense and nervous. Likewise, chronic insomniacs find that exercise relieves their anxieties and induces healthy fatigue.

The reduction of anxiety through exercise also is helpful in treating some patients with emotional problems.

We know from psychological testing that a patient's self-image improves as the result of systematic exercise. This in itself may be a great help in treating certain emotional problems.

Several psychiatrists have reported good results using

exercise as an adjunct to therapy in patients with certain psychiatric problems, particularly states of mild depression. One of my psychiatric correspondents expressed the thought that a "physically fit patient responds more readily to psychotherapy."

Exercise has recently been employed in the treatment of chronic alcoholics in clinics in Sweden. The initial observations are encouraging, but it is too early to draw conclusions.

A few readers of *Aerobics* claimed that exercise helped, and in some cases, relieved them of their problem with migraine headaches. I can't scientifically document such a statement and therefore report it only as an observation.

The embarrassing problem of incontinence (passing urine when coughing or sneezing) frequently occurs in women after several pregnancies. Some women have written claiming that this condition either disappeared or improved in response to exercise. Apparently the improvement in muscle tone through walking and running enabled these women to regain better control over their bladders.

Many older people have informed me that the arthritis in their legs and back improved with aerobic training. To the contrary, others claim that their arthritis was aggravated by exercise. So the evidence for the beneficial effect of aerobics is still inconclusive.

The whole field of exercise therapy is now in a state of transition from faddism to scientific legitimacy. Hardly a month passes without the publication of a significant new report on the numerous medical applications of exercise. As research expands, I hope that it will be possible to formulate specific aerobic routines for a variety of therapeutic uses.

9: Mostly About Women

I TEND TO disagree with the fellow who first remarked that "beauty is only skin-deep." Quite to the contrary, I believe that beauty in a woman is a reflection of her total well-being, of her basic health and vitality.

It depends, of course, on what you mean by beauty. At one time in our history, it was considered very elegant for a woman to look as though she were in imminent danger of physical collapse. Later on beauty grew more robust. A good-looking woman was supposed to be "pleasantly plump," (her plumpness size) being regarded as a sign of prosperity and good social standing.

Today's ideas are different. The emancipation of women in the twentieth century has given rise to a new ideal of feminine beauty. Today we admire women whose appearance shows that they are competent and capable—women with lean but strong bodies moving with the natural grace of a healthy creature.

This kind of beauty is definitely not just skin-deep. It involves posture, gait, and personality—it is the assurance and the glow that springs from fitness, alertness, and high spirits.

Feminine appeal, of course, is something every man judges for himself. But many, I think, will agree with me that a trim shape and graceful movement add as much to a girl's attractiveness as a pretty face. What really counts is charm—that subtle mixture compounded of both physical and mental attributes that is reflected in stance, motion, manner and voice.

All this may seem a long way from aerobics, but really it isn't. Because exercise changes a person both physically and mentally, it directly affects those factors of physique and personality that are the secret of feminine charm.

I am not peddling miracles. Obviously, exercise alone cannot completely transform you and your personality but, quite aside from physical improvements, exercise may help you to gain self-confidence and give you a feeling of calm complaisance. Granted, exercise cannot—and should not—make you a basically different person. But it can—and should—help you make the most of what you have and what you are.

The kind of personal attractiveness that comes from fitness and health is by no means confined to young women only. When you see a woman of 50 looking like 30, or a woman of 60 looking—and acting—like 40, chances are that she is one of the growing number of middle-aged women who prolong their youthfulness by preventive health care including regular exercise. Their outward signs of age-defying youthfulness—the straight back, taut, smooth skin on face, neck, arms and legs, and supple muscle contours—are evidence that these women don't spend all their spare time sitting before a TV set, moping over their lost youth.

I recall with pleasure the exhilarating sight of a woman, well past 40, giving her daughter a hard time on the tennis court. Both were good players, but the older woman was faster on her feet. Repeatedly rushing the net, she gained an advantage from her agility that enabled her to beat her daughter, who was less than half her age.

Later when she joined us on the club terrace, looking every bit as handsome and vigorous as her own daughter, I complimented her on her game. "Oh," she laughed, "nowadays parents have to keep up with their children."

That is an important point, in more than one way. I am convinced that if parents and their children found active companionship in sports, there would be less of a "generation gap." Shared physical activity is a common ground on which to build mutual understanding.

Recent medical research has given us new insights into the process of aging, and there is evidence indicating that premature aging is accelerated by inactivity. True, other factors are involved, especially heredity and diet. But physical stagnation due to lack of exercise seems to be a major factor in premature aging.

Aerobics therefore has a special significance for the older woman. By prolonging her good looks and vitality, aerobics can help a middle-aged woman attain what may well be her happiest years.

WEIGHT AND FIGURE

Even more than men, women have fallen victims to our sedentary era. At one time, women got a fair amount of exercise just by working in the garden and walking to the grocery store. Few women today tend a kitchen garden; the vegetables are frozen, and you order them by phone.

This avoidance of physical effort extends to every phase of life. Since two-car families are now the suburban rule, the only walking many women do is in parking lots. And city women tell me that, times being what they are, they find it safer not to go out after working hours. Increasingly, women have been deprived of walking and other natural forms of exercise. No wonder so many of them gain weight and lose their figures.

Modern women, therefore, have a particular need of a systematic exercise program, and aerobics has helped countless women take off extra pounds and inches.

Of all the women who have told me of their experience with aerobics, Bertha Whitson is my favorite. She lived in our neighborhood and everyone noticed her, but not in the way a woman likes to be noticed.

Bert was 5' 2" and had a sweet and pretty face. Few people ever looked at it. They were too busy staring at—or away from—her excessively overweight frame.

Bert read about aerobics in the *Reader's Digest*. Realizing the need for a change, she asked her physician about starting into an exercise program.

After making sure that her obesity was not due to a medical problem, he said: "What you need is a combination of both diet and exercise. The diet gets rid of excess weight. And the exercise keeps you from gaining it right back after you stop dieting."

Bert was willing to try anything. She went on a moderate diet and began exercising with a kind of brave determination I have rarely seen in anyone.

At first she could hardly move. Running was out of the question. Her thighs were so thick that it was difficult for her to move her legs back and forth in a straight line.

Yet despite these handicaps, and the enormous effort they entailed, Bert started walking every day. Gradually she increased the distance she walked. By the end of six months, she was walking ten miles a day—five miles during the morning, and another five miles in the evening.

Her daily route led her past the football field of the local high school, where her regular appearance was eagerly awaited by some ungentlemanly young athletes who hooted at her laborious progress. But after a few weeks, the boys' attitude changed. Something in Bert's undaunted persistence won their respect. "I felt like a turtle in a turtle race," recalls Bert, "what with all the bystanders cheering and egging me on."

Bystanders weren't the only ones cheering for Bert. Her husband was delighted by both the physical and emotional changes in her. Within one year of daily walking and moderate dieting she lost 50 pounds. Instead of size 18, she now wears size ten. Once again, her husband saw the small, graceful girl he had married.

Not only did she regain her looks; her former sprightliness and good humor returned also. This change of mood partly reflected her pride in her own accomplishment, and the pleasure any woman feels in being physically attractive. But her high spirits also stemmed from the fact that regular exercise gave her more energy.

"I never really lived through the day, when I was so heavy," Bert admits. "I just dragged myself through it. By the time my husband came home at night, I was exhausted and disgusted. Now I have the energy to feel alive in the evening. And I'm better company for my husband."

I never think of Bert as just a case history. I'm frankly touched by this woman's determination. If there were more like her, there would be a lot more happy women and happy families in this country.

My own wife, Millie, also relies on aerobics to keep in condition and to keep her shape. Looking at her now—a trim 5'5", 120 pounds—nobody would believe she ever had a weight problem. But she likes Southern style cooking, and has a yen for second helpings. Not surprisingly, she tended to be a little heavier than she wanted to be—by about fifteen pounds or so.

Being a tidy person with a natural concern about her appearance, Millie used to go on crash diets, eating only dry salads and hardboiled eggs, with nothing for breakfast except a cup of black coffee. By such a drastic means, she'd drop in weight fairly rapidly.

Then she'd get ravenously hungry, quit her diet and gain it all back. Exercise, I knew, could help her with her problem. I asked her to start jogging with me, but with my longer stride and better physical condition, I usually got far ahead of her. I had to give myself a handicap. We finally hit on the idea of taking our young daughter along with us. Pushing her in the stroller slowed me down enough so Millie could keep up and it gave me an excellent work out!

Five times a week we jogged, alternately walking and running, up to 1.5 miles. At first, Millie would run only on the downhill stretches, walking the remainder of the way. But gradually, as she got into condition, the walking segments got shorter and shorter. Now she runs the entire distance, and covers the 1.5 miles in just over 12 minutes. This earns her 6 points per run or 30 points per five-day week.

She's eating normally now—with second helpings. But thanks to the exercise, she doesn't put on weight. She's particularly pleased that exercise accomplished what diet alone never could: taking inches off her hips and thighs.

It also reduced her resting heart rate. One night, before Millie started exercising, we counted each other's heart beat just before going to sleep. Mine was 45 beats per minute. Hers was 85.

"I don't want to wear out so much faster than you do!" she said.

Actually, there is no medical evidence that a person has a fixed number of heartbeats per lifetime and that a faster pulse uses up his quota that much sooner. Yet there is no doubt that a slower resting heart rate is less work for the heart.

At any rate, after Millie began exercising regularly, her resting heart rate dropped to less than 60. Her attitude toward exercise is different from mine. I enjoy it. She doesn't. But she keeps at it just the same.

"I still don't really like running," she confessed to me not long ago. "I just look at it as something I do for my health. Like brushing my teeth."

"You mean you don't get any pleasure from it at all?" I asked.

"Oh, sure," she replied. "Every step of the way I think

how I'm going to fit into that size eight dress and how good that cherry pie is going to taste."

Some women go on crash diets to lose weight, but from a medical viewpoint this is certainly not advisable. With a crash diet, which is basically a form of fasting, you may lose as much muscle as fat. True, it takes off pounds and inches, but it certainly doesn't contribute to your fitness. To the contrary, on such a strict diet you'll soon notice the onset of weakness and fatigue.

Yet a moderate diet combined with exercise lets you lose fat and weight while at the same time it strengthens your muscles. And by increasing your aerobic capacity you gain new energy reserves as you reduce. Instead of feeling weak and nervous as a result of your diet, the addition of exercise makes you feel fit and vigorous.

Women are usually surprised when I tell them that exercise also can change their shape even without changing their weight. It lets them take off inches without taking off pounds.

"How can you get smaller without getting lighter?" they ask. The answer is that exercise changes the fat–muscle ratio. Since muscle tissue is a lot more dense than fat, the same weight takes up less space.

While most women use aerobics to take off inches, I know of at least one who put on some inches just where she wanted them.

"I didn't like the looks of my bird legs," writes Mrs. Martha Frank from Lake Village, Arkansas. "I wanted a pair of legs I wouldn't have to hide in slacks.

"So, I started on a running program—on a seldom used blacktop road near the house and barn. I'm 43 years old, and now my family calls me 'Supersport.' I had a little trouble at first with sore arches, but now I'm doing 1.5 miles in 14 minutes and 30 seconds and hope to work my way up into the top fitness category.

"I knew I needed the exercise. I spend most of my time sitting in the truck, driving to cattle auctions—and on weekends sitting at the desk doing the paper work. It made a great difference in the way I feel. And, oh yes, those legs really shaped up. . . ."

Most women frankly admit that they exercise mainly for the sake of their looks. "It makes you feel just fantastic," writes one of my correspondents, "to receive flattering remarks about your youthful looking figure."

Vanity? Not really. The way a woman looks has a great deal to do with the way she feels—and how others feel about her. It's not just a matter of catching or keeping a husband. The attitude of other women toward her, her effectiveness in the community, her chances in a career, even the respect of her children depend to some degree on her appearance. Perhaps it is unfortunate that a woman's total personality is so strongly linked to her appearance. Yet, undeniably, it's part of our culture. Every woman senses it. So to be concerned about her figure is not just vanity but solid good sense.

The way it works out, women earn a double payoff from aerobics: they go on the program to improve their looks, and they get fitness and health as fringe benefits.

PREGNANCY AND AFTER

The greatest physical challenge the average woman faces during her life is childbearing. Far too many women are unprepared for the muscular strain of pregnancy and childbirth. By toning up the abdominal and back muscles, aerobics enables women to carry and deliver their infants more easily and swiftly regain their figures afterward. Besides, the overall improvement of health may have a favorable effect on the child's prenatal development. And it may reduce the danger of circulatory and cardiac complications for the mother.

The muscular conditioning obtained through aerobics also helps avoid some of the painful aftereffects of pregnancy and childbirth.

"Oh, my aching back!" is one of the most common complaints a doctor hears from women after pregnancy and childbirth. Even very young mothers often suffer severe and chronic back pains.

In an article published in the *Journal of the American Medical Association,* it was reported that a lack of exercise in women 18–23 years of age was a frequent cause of backache following pregnancy.

Ideally, a woman should be in good condition before the onset of pregnancy. But she can start into an exercise program during pregnancy, if she consults her obstetrician. She may have a condition that would make exercise inadvisable. Normally it is possible for women to continue their regular aerobic exercise program up to the sixth month of pregnancy. After that, exercise should be less strenuous. A simple walking program may be the most suitable during the last three months.

Of course, there are exceptions to every rule. One of my correspondents in Ann Arbor, Michigan, kept right on jogging throughout her pregnancy. "Even during the ninth month," she writes, "I kept up my daily routine. A 12-minute morning jog, and another 12 minutes jogging late in the evening. All with my obstetrician's approval, of course.

"As a result I felt absolutely marvelous all through my pregnancy and had no difficulty keeping my weight down. My doctor wanted me to do this because he was considering the possibility of a Caesarean section.

"The Caesarean section was not necessary and due to the jogging, I still have my waistline and a flat tummy—not the deflated beach ball I thought I'd end up with."

And then she ended her letter with an amusing comment. "But you know what, Dr. Cooper?—my baby seems to have an unusual fondness for being bounced on the knee!"

Even if your obstetrician decides that exercise is not advisable for you during pregnancy, he will probably permit you to resume exercise after the birth of your child. Any of the aerobic conditioning programs will tone up slack muscles, and help give you your old shape back.

MEN AND WOMEN—THE DIFFERENCE

Whatever may be said of women's hearts in other respects, medically speaking they have less of a problem with coronary disease than men—at least before the age of 40. Coronary heart disease is rare in women of childbearing age. After menopause, though, women begin to lose this advantage. Consequently, a woman's exercise program should be geared to this natural timetable.

This brings us to the difference in exercise requirements for women as compared with men. Since younger women are somewhat immune to heart and blood vessel disease, they do not share a man's need for aerobics as a basic life preserver. Consequently, they don't need to build up as many points as men. Probably, 20–24 points per week is enough. But after menopause, when women begin to lose their natural resistance to cardiovascular disease, they should definitely work up to at least 24 points per week to gain the full preventive effect.

The distance requirements for the 12-minute test for women (page 30) are based on accumulating 24 points per week. With this level of activity, the age adjusted requirements should be achieved easily.

CALISTHENICS FOR WOMEN

Calisthenics develop certain qualities of special interest to women, particularly graceful coordination of movement. For younger women I frequently suggest the addition of calisthenics to their aerobic routine. With calisthenics enhancing the grace of movement and aerobics providing basic fitness and reserve energy, it's a winning combination.

Of the many kinds of calisthenics, I particularly recommend five basic exercises that have been developed for women members of the United States Marine Corps:

1. *Trunk circling:* Stand with your legs apart and twist the upper part of your body alternately to the left and the right, rotating mainly from the waist.

2. *Toe touching:* with your legs fairly close together, bend from the waist to touch your toes with outstretched arms. If you cannot reach all the way down with your knees straight, bend your knees slightly.

3. *Side leg-raise:* Lie on the floor on your side and raise the leg from the hip, then lower it again. Repeat about ten times, then turn to the other side and raise and lower the other leg ten times.

4. *Sit-ups:* Lie on the floor, on your back, with your knees bent. Raise the trunk to a sitting position without the help of arms, then lie down again *slowly*. Start with about ten repetitions. (Sit-ups are traditionally attempted with legs stretched out flat against the floor. I advise against this because the stress on the knees and back may cause pain and even injury. It is far safer to bend the knees slightly during sit-up exercises.)

5. *Side bends:* Stand with your feet apart and extend your arms above your head with fingertips touching. Bend slowly sideways from the waist as far as possible. Keep your arms straight and don't bend your elbows. Remain bent sideways for several seconds. Then straighten up and make a similar bend to the other side, again remaining in a bent position for a few seconds.

Working up to 20 repetitions of each of these five forms of calisthenic, in combination with aerobic exercise, will give younger women an optimum exercise blend.

I have been asked why I specifically recommend calisthenics for women but not for men. Some people draw the inference that I am against calisthenics for men. This is definitely not so. A man may gain from calisthenics the same benefits as a woman. Also, he tends to build certain muscles that otherwise might not be fully developed. But what men need most—heart protection and overall fitness—calisthenics alone can't provide.

Put it this way: Calisthenics are fine as long as they are done *in addition to* rather than *in place of* one of the primary aerobics exercises.

SPECIAL PROBLEMS

Women often ask whether they should exercise during their menstrual period. It depends on the individual case. Women suffering from cramps find exercise extremely uncomfortable. Common sense alone tells them to skip exercise during those days. But, in principle, there is no reason why a woman should stop exercising during her menstrual period, except when it proves painful.

Women frequently develop painful or swollen muscles and joints in response to jogging or stationary running. One possible reason is that in their younger years they do not engage in sports as regularly as men. As a result, their muscles may not be adequately prepared for vigorous aerobic conditioning.

But this problem does not usually persist. After a few days of light exercise or complete rest, the pain tends to disappear. In those rare cases where muscle pains persist with exercise, the best thing to do is simply prolong the conditioning program. Progress very slowly. If necessary, repeat each week so that the muscles get a better chance to adapt themselves to the increasing work load. Another possibility is to alternate different kinds of exercise. Suppose your ankles get sore after stationary running. Switch to cycling for a while to give your ankles a different kind of workout. This enables you to continue your progressive aerobic program without aggravating a joint problem.

Some of the special problems encountered by women aren't physical at all. They're purely a matter of attitude. One of the WAF's in the Air Force aerobics test project seemed obviously reluctant during the daily workouts I supervised. When I asked her about this she responded with a pleasant smile: "It's not ladylike to run!"

"Well, is it ladylike for a woman to participate in any type of exercise?" I asked her.

The point I was trying to get through her pretty head is that outmoded notions of femininity just no longer apply. In an age when young women may join military organizations, win Olympic medals, and compete with men on terms of equality in almost any field, we had better get rid of our notions about what's ladylike and what isn't. I can't imagine why healthful exercise should be considered improper or unsuitable.

In the course of administering aerobics programs, I've seen women as eager and determined as any man in pursuit of physical fitness. Yet I have also observed that some women have a talent for self-pity. They slow down as soon as the exercise gets the least bit strenuous. This ruins any accurate comparison between field and laboratory testing. Specifically, the field test/treadmill correlation for women was only 0.57 as compared with 0.9 for men. Again, it appears to be a matter of motivation and attitude.

I know of at least one woman who certainly has no motivation problems and who has done more than anyone to dispel the myth that women can't do as well as men when it comes to athletics. In the sports world, she is known as Super Sue. Her real name is Susan Bailey, 25 years old, and mother of two children. Her hobby is long-distance running.

Sue has run as far as 38 miles nonstop. In 1968, she entered the national YMCA 3000-mile marathon as the only girl in the 24-man 1-woman team from her home town of Canton, Ohio. The Canton team dropped their national record from 6.5 days to a phenomenal 4.5 days, and Sue contributed 208 miles to the 3000 mile total—the third highest contribution made by any individual team member.

You would think that a woman of this kind would look tough and musclebound. But when I show pictures of Sue at my lectures, there is always an appreciative "Ah!" from the audience. No wonder—for Sue is as pretty and graceful a girl as you will ever see—living proof that sports and true feminine charm go well together.

Since most exercise research has been conducted on men, we still do not have quite enough information on the special needs and problems of exercising women. I would be grateful for any data my readers can contribute on the subject of fitness testing and exercise programs for women.

OVER 40

That life begins at 40 is hardly true. But it certainly doesn't stop there either. I wish more women could convince themselves that the age of 40, or 50, or 60, is not some magic dividing line beyond which nothing good ever happens.

Modern medicine can successfully deal with many of the physical symptoms of aging, minimizing their discomfort. Just within the past few years great strides have been made in this area, and exercise is of considerable importance to a woman who wants to keep young regardless of age.

Quite aside from the physical benefits of exercise, post-menopausal women get a special psychological lift from a regular exercise program. Too often women in that age group suffer a kind of melancholy or mental slump. They go into a depression, becoming cranky and difficult to live with.

I have seen such women improve remarkably through regular exercise. Just why aerobics has the effect of a psychological tonic, I cannot say with scientific precision. But the final effect is obvious. Physical well-being due to regular exercise, plus awareness of improved appearance, evidently gives a needed lift to a woman's mental attitude.

I encountered a striking example of this when we asked the wives of some retired military personnel to join in an aerobics program at our laboratory. About two months after the start of this project I received a visit from a retired officer. He came right to the point and said simply: "I want to thank you for really helping our marriage."

His wife, he told me, had become quite erratic at the age of 48, suffering unpredictable emotional ups and downs. "One day she'd feel all keyed up—all smiles and chatter. The next day she'd sulk and hardly say a word. Sometimes she'd have sudden bitter outbursts, complaining how our lives had been wasted, and how I had robbed her of every chance of happiness. She had illusions of poverty, even though we live quite comfortably. Then she'd go out on a spending spree. She even started interfering in the married lives of our two children. The whole thing was irrational. I didn't know how to deal with it, but I knew it couldn't go on that way."

Then came the turning point. A friend told her about our aerobics club for women. Prompted by her feelings of loneliness, the woman probably would have joined any group that asked her. Luckily, this happened to be just what she needed. Under the stimulus of regular exercise, a set goal, new companions and, above all, improved physical health, she regained her emotional balance. "I think it occurred without her realizing what was happening," her husband said. "She simply went back to normal."

I am not saying that aerobics can be relied on as a cure for emotional disturbances. Obviously, most situations of this type need psychiatric treatment. I am merely reporting an observation: Some women suffering post-menopausal depression have been greatly helped by participation in a regular exercise program.

In one respect, older women should practice special caution during exercise. After menopause, they frequently suffer a condition known as osteoporosis. This causes loss of calcium from the bones, making them brittle. Consequently, older women are more likely to suffer bone fractures. I therefore caution older women about stationary running or rope skipping since these exercises put high stress on the bones of the foot and lower leg.

INDOOR EXERCISE

Women often are housebound. They have to watch the kids, clean the house, cook, do the washing and wait for the delivery man. Their chances to go outdoors for exercise are often limited, and quite aside from the restriction of climate, many women hesitate to go out running in the street.

"People think I'm crazy. They gawk at me," complains a Baltimore housewife who tried jogging around her neighborhood. In contrast to European cities, our own metropolitan areas suffer a drastic shortage of safe, usable parkland and walking paths. As a result, many people—especially women —depend on indoor exercise to earn aerobic points.

Women also like indoor exercise because they can do it without really having to concentrate on it. "I do my stationary running right in front of the TV set," writes an Idaho girl. "That way I get my points, I'm entertained, and the time passes rapidly."

Among the most efficient indoor exercises are stationary running, skipping rope, climbing stairs, stationary cycling and running on a treadmill. A few brief comments on these exercises now, and then I will discuss them in more detail in Chapter Ten.

STATIONARY RUNNING

To avoid foot and ankle trouble, wear cushioned-soled shoes and run on a soft surface, preferably on a thick rug. Pick your knees up in front lifting your feet at least 8 inches off the floor and run at the rate of 80–90 steps per minute. If that seems too fast for you, try 70–80 steps.

To check your speed, count every time your left foot hits the floor. Do this for 15 seconds, then multiply by 4. This gives you your step-per-minute figure.

Some women like to do their stationary running in time to music. It helps keep the rhythm steady and reduces boredom. The trick is finding a record with the proper beat and one that maintains a steady rhythm for a long enough period. There are some jogging records on the market that can be used very effectively in a stationary running program.

ROPE SKIPPING

In some ways, rope skipping is an ideal indoor exercise. It not only gives you the same aerobic benefits as stationary running, but it also provides additional exercise for the muscles of arms, shoulders, and upper torso. This may help to improve a woman's appearance, by toning up the muscles in the arms, shoulders and chest, giving added support to the bust.

What's more, rope skipping is not as likely to cause ankle and leg pain and swelling as stationary running because it lessens the impact of the feet against the floor.

You can skip rope in four different ways: 1) jumping with both feet together; 2) alternating left and right foot; 3) jumping up and down on one leg only; 4) stepping over the rope, one foot at a time.

My recommendation is to use modes one and two. Of course, rope skipping can be done at widely different speeds, from a very slow rate to the fast routine used by professional boxers as part of their conditioning. I recommend about 70–80 steps per minute—the same rate as in stationary running.

Under these conditions, rope skipping has the same point value as stationary running.

STAIR CLIMBING

"Who do you suppose earns more aerobic points: a woman who keeps running up and down the first three steps of her staircase for five minutes or a woman who runs up and down several flights of stairs for the same length of time?"

I threw that question at one of my lab assistants as a teaser. His answer was absolutely correct: the woman running only three steps at a time earns more points. The woman running up and down several flights loses some of the aerobic benefit because the down trip allows her body time to recover. The three-step course provides more continuity of effort—an essential factor in earning aerobic points.

The point value of stair climbing as well as the use of stationary bicycles, self-propelled and motorized treadmills will be discussed in detail in Chapter Ten.

While it is usually women who are chiefly interested in indoor exercise, there's no reason why men can't join them.

Certainly one of the most important things a woman can do for her husband is to motivate him to join her in regular exercise. Just recently, I received a letter from a Wisconsin housewife describing such a joint venture.

"I love my husband," she writes, "and I want to keep him with me as long as possible—that's why I persuaded him to exercise with me. During the winter we can't run outdoors. So we laid out a track in our basement: Sure, it's short. It takes 80 laps 'to the mile. But when my husband and I do it together, it's fun."

In their domestic lives, women often become the victims of routine. Many of them lack the challenges that men face in their work. For a woman whose home is her career, the years can become a long, losing battle against boredom. Aerobics has proved to be a turning point in the lives of many such women. Getting on the program marks for them the point of a new departure. They shed boredom and become alert and responsive again. The vitality women gain from upgrading their fitness sometimes opens the door to many other interests, giving their whole existence new dimensions of meaning.

A POSTSCRIPT ON CHILDREN

Every mother teaches her children how to wash, brush their teeth, and perform other habits of personal care and hygiene. Training children to exercise is just as vital to their future health.

In this respect, we, as a nation, don't do a very good job in bringing up our children. Physical fitness is widely neglected by the younger generation, as proved by the rejection rate from the armed forces. As much as 40 percent of all eligible draftees don't measure up to the minimum fitness standards for military service. In terms of national health, this is clearly an emergency situation. Early parental teaching of the value of exercise would be a most effective countermeasure.

Little is yet known about the specific exercise needs of children in the six to 16 age group, and I am trying to obtain additional information in this field. I shall be grateful to any parent, grade school teacher, or junior high school athletics instructor, who can provide me with pertinent observations regarding 12-minute or other field test data, particularly before and after a conditioning program.

Yet some basic facts have been uncovered. Dr. Ernst Jokl, director of the Exercise Research Laboratories of the University of Kentucky, tested 4000 children aged six to 18, by checking their performance in a 600-yard run. He found that girls reach maximum fitness during puberty, but soon lose it again unless their fitness level is maintained by exercise. This may account for the fact that girl swimmers of Olympic caliber are usually in their early teens.

Boys achieve a high-level endurance capacity between the ages of 18 and 21. Not surprisingly, our fastest milers are young men in this age bracket. Marathon champions are usually a little older—24–28 years of age.

Even very young children are sometimes capable of surprising feats of endurance. For example, at the Dipsia Marathon, a 6.8-mile race held annually in California, a five-year-old girl entered the race and finished a very respectable 441st among 900 entries. Among the adult contestants outrun by the little girl were both her parents.

However, I do not advise any kind of endurance exercise for children before the age of six. If such small children enjoy the simpler forms of calisthenics, they might practice them for a few minutes each day. This will give them agility and coordination. Especially if they are encouraged to do these simple exercises while their mother does her aerobics, children form a positive attitude toward physical training. They learn early in life that fitness can be fun.

From the age of six onward, children may participate in low-level aerobic exercise, though the quantitative norms for small children yet remain to be worked out. Running, cycling and swimming are excellent for children, but parents should see to it that children do not exhaust themselves in such activities. Often their abundant energy tempts children beyond their endurance. A parent's common sense should be a safeguard against overexertion.

EXERCISE AT SCHOOL

For children of school age, regular exercise should be part of their school curriculum. In October 1968, the American Academy of Pediatrics issued a set of guidelines for athletics for elementary school children. It is an excellent paper which I strongly recommend to school principals and physical education teachers. In particular, I agree with the academy's objection to competitive team sports for young children. Too much emotional stress is associated with such competition. In particular, the Academy cautions against "undesirable corollaries to organized competitive athletics, such as excessive publicity, pep squads, commercial promoting, victory celebrations, paid admissions, inappropriate spectator behavior, high-pressure public contests and exploitation of children in any form."

The child should learn to enjoy sports and exercise for their own sake—not for commercial or competitive reasons.

The importance of regular exercise in school has been shown by the fact that California school children have enjoyed a much higher fitness level than children from most other states. This was probably attributable to the fact that they had a state law requiring a scheduled daily exercise for students in all grades. Unfortunately, in 1968, the law was modified to allow more flexibility in scheduling of exercise periods, eliminating the mandatory daily requirement.

A high school science teacher of my acquaintance once told me that, in his experience, youngsters active in athletics tend to do better in their classwork. I knew that he himself was an avid sports fan, and so I dismissed his observation as a reflection of his own attitudes and prejudices. To imply that school athletics were directly beneficial to academic work seemed a little far-fetched.

Yet several studies with high school and college students have shown that those students who are more physically fit consistently make better grades. It isn't realistic to believe that physically fit students are more intelligent. But that they are probably more alert and receptive may be the reason that they make better grades.

In view of this apparent link between physical and mental achievement, it is all the more regrettable that our school systems offer so little in the way of physical conditioning.

"Many children in the United States," says Dr. Stanley L. Harrison of the American Academy of Pediatrics, "although healthy and well-nourished, are still in relatively poor physical condition simply because they live in a civilization on wheels. They ride to school in the bus or the family car.

And physical education in school too often consists of just a softball game, which provides a minimum of strenuous exertion."

This is an area where parents, and mothers in particular, can make their influence felt. Through organizations like the PTA, they can insist on properly managed exercise programs in the schools, especially at the grade school and junior high school level. A young mother in Houston wrote to tell me she was running for the school board and one of her campaign promises was to replace baseball in grade school with aerobics exercise. More power to her!

No school program, however well conceived, can in itself offset the damaging influence on a child of our physically passive way of life. It's clearly up to the family, and the mother in particular, to bring up the children with a keen awareness of the physical requirements of a healthful life. She can do a great service to her children by implanting the idea that exercise is not just "something you have to do" but a lifelong source of pleasure.

10: Indoor Exercising

WITH THE WIDESPREAD lack of public recreation facilities in our cities, our inadequate parks, crowded sidewalks, and the absence of walking paths or country lanes suitable for extended walking or running, I often hear the complaint, "I just don't have any place to exercise." Usually this is followed by the question, "What can I do in my own home?"

I have received hundreds of letters with questions related to home exercise: How many points can I earn by stationary cycling? Must I subtract point value for walking on a self-propelled treadmill? Does it make any difference if the treadmill is set at an incline? And—the most commonly asked question on indoor exercise—How many points for walking up a flight of stairs?

The purpose of this chapter is to deal with questions of this kind and to help you plan an aerobics conditioning program you can complete without ever leaving your home.

STATIONARY RUNNING (MODIFIED)

One of the basic indoor aerobics exercises is stationary running. It has, however, several drawbacks. It is hard on the ankles, and most people find it boring. Consequently, they are looking for variations in this tedious routine.

You might, to add variety to your exercise program, use a single step—preferably a cushioned step to prevent slipping. Start with both feet on the floor and step up, bringing boht feet onto the step (one after the other—do not jump), then return your feet to the floor, one at a time. Do this rapidly, at the rate of 30–40 full cycles per minute. The aerobic point value for this type of exercise is as follows:

POINT VALUE FOR EXERCISE USING A SINGLE STEP

(Approximately 7 inches in height)

Stepping Rate (per Min)	Time (Min)	Points
30	6:30	1½
	9:45	2¼
	13:00	3
35	6:00	2
	9:00	3
	12:00	4
40	5:00	2½
	7:30	3¾
	10:00	5

Another variant of stationary running is to use three steps and run up and down the steps, turning around at the top so that you always face forward. Do this at the rate of about 20 complete trips per minute. The point value for this exercise is roughly equivalent to the point value for stationary running at a rate of 70–80 steps per minute. At a rate of 25–30 complete trips per minute, it is equivalent to stationary running at 80–90 steps per minute.

STAIR CLIMBING (AEROBICALLY)

"On my way to work, I walk up several flights of stairs every morning. It takes me about two minutes. How many points do I get?"

My questioner was quite disappointed when I told him that he gets no points at all. Even walking eight to ten flights or more doesn't really help to condition the cardiovascular system because the time interval is too short. True, it may leave you breathless—because you have built up a big oxygen debt during your climb. But the climb just didn't last long enough for the training effect to set in.

Yet there is a way to make good use of a single flight of stairs for aerobic conditioning. Making complete trips up and down that flight can be an excellent way to earn aerobic points. You can even carry some weight with you to increase the point value of this exercise.

For people who find this a convenient exercise method, I have developed the following point-value charts for stair-climbing with and without a load.

POINT VALUE FOR STAIR CLIMBING USING A SINGLE FLIGHT OF STAIRS

(10 Steps; 6–7 inches in height; 25–30° incline)

Round trips (Average Number per Min)	Duration (Min)	Points Without Load	Points (With 10 lb. Load)
6	6:30	1½	2
	9:45	2¼	3
	13:00	3	4
7	6:00	2	2½
	9:00	3	3¾
	12:00	4	5
8	5:30	2½	3
	8:15	3¾	4½
	11:00	5	6
9	4:30	2¾	3¼
	6:45	4¼	4½
	9:00	5¾	6¾
10	4:00	3¼	3¾
	6:00	4¾	5½
	8:00	6½	7½

STATIONARY BICYCLES

These increasingly popular home exercise devices come in various price ranges with different design features.

1. Low cost models ($25–35): No brake resistance device, no speed or mileage indicator. Usually of limited value in aerobic conditioning programs since it is impossible to measure performance accurately enough to follow the progressive exercise charts.

2. Medium-cost models ($75–120): Equipped with speed and mileage indicators and brake resistance devices—everything you need to follow the aerobic charts accurately.

3 Moderately expensive models (about $350): In this category I should like to single out a Swedish exercise bicycle with speed and mileage indicators and a *calibrated* brake resistance device—excellent for either testing or conditioning programs.

4. Expensive models (about $650): These models are motor-driven. You don't supply the energy by pedaling. Hence they are of little value for aerobic conditioning unless you compensate for the work contributed by the motor. You can buy an auxiliary meter that shows how much energy you are expending.

5. Very expensive models (about $900): A stationary bicycle with built-in heart rate monitor and "electronic coach." This provides hills and valleys along the simulated ride by means of pre-programmed variations of brake resistance. You can watch your heart rate on a monitor, making sure that it does not go too high. This is an excellent bike for rehabilitation programs, gyms, YMCAs, and health clubs, though it may be too expensive for the average home user.

Whatever stationary bicycle you may buy, follow these rules as you use it in your aerobic conditioning program:

1. Cycle at an indicated speed of 15–20 miles per hour. Some bikes have a tachometer instead of a speedometer. In that case, keep a cycling rate of 60–80 rpm.

2. Watch your mileage indicator and cycle the distance specified in the charts for one of the progressive cycling programs (see Chapter Six). Generally, I recommend starting with the Category I program.

3. Add enough brake resistance so that immediately after the conclusion of the exercise your heart rate is slightly in excess of the age-adjusted rates given below:

Age (Years)	Heart Rate (beats per minute)
Under 30	160
30–34	155
35–39	150
40–44	145
45–49	145
50–54	140
55–59	140
60–64	135
65+	130

(To check your heart rate, count the beats for the first ten seconds after exercise and then multiply by six).

If you follow these simple rules, you can get on your bicycle and ride your way to physical fitness without ever leaving home.

TREADMILLS

Judging by my correspondence, there is even greater interest in treadmills than in stationary bicycles. As to your choice of a treadmill, again you have a variety of models in different price ranges:

1. Inexpensive ($99–285): These treadmills are muscle-powered and can be used effectively if you can learn to walk or run on them without holding on to the side rails. This may be difficult since the treadmills were not designed for this manner of use. Some models provide a built-in incline, which increases aerobic value, as I shall explain later.

2. Medium-priced ($385): A new model available in this price group is motor-driven with a speed selection of three, four, or five miles per hour, which covers the range of walking and slow jogging. Elevate the front end with blocks and you can operate the treadmill at an incline to earn more aerobic points. The design of this treadmill is very good.

3. Expensive ($1000–1500): Motor driven treadmills in this price range offer variable speeds up to 7–8 miles per hour, which is fast enough for most people. Also they provide a built-in adjustable incline. Such treadmills are highly effective indoor exercise devices.

4. Very expensive ($3500 or more): These are research models, similar to the one I use in my laboratory. The speed is variable from 1.5 to 25 miles per hour and the incline can be adjusted from zero to 40 percent. It is an excellent device but prohibitive in cost for the average home user.

Whatever treadmill you may buy, you must follow certain basic rules. Leave the treadmill at zero inclination and use either the Category I running or walking program and follow it exactly as if you were exercising outdoors. If you want to get more points, add some incline. As you can see from the chart below, walking or running up an incline is worth considerably more aerobic points than exercising with no incline.

POINT VALUE FOR WALKING AND RUNNING ONE MILE ON A
TREADMILL SET AT VARIOUS INCLINES

TREADMILL Speed (MPH)	Mile Time (Min)	Incline (% grade)				
		0%	5%	10%	15%	
10	6:00	6	7	9	—	
7.5	8:00	5	6	7	10	
6	10:00	4	5	6	7	
5	12:00	3	4	5	6	Points
4.14	14:30	2	4	5	6	
3	20:00	1	1.5	2.5	3	
2.5	25:00	0	1	1.5	2	
		0°	3°	6°	9°	

Incline (degrees)

You can use a motorized treadmill in still another way, providing it is equipped with a speedometer. You leave your treadmill at zero incline and set it at a certain speed. Then stay on the treadmill at that speed for the required number of minutes. The point value of such exercise can easily be determined from the following chart:

POINTS FOR WALKING OR RUNNING ONE MILE ON A
MOTORIZED TREADMILL (No Incline)

Mile Time	Treadmill Speed	Points
6:00 Min	10 MPH	6
6:30 Min	9¼ MPH	6
7:00 Min	8½ MPH	5
7:30 Min	8 MPH	5
8:00 Min	7½ MPH	5
8:30 Min	7 MPH	4
9:00 Min	6⅔ MPH	4
9:30 Min	6⅓ MPH	4
10:00 Min	6 MPH	4
12:00 Min	5 MPH	3
13:30 Min	4½ MPH	2
15:00 Min	4 MPH	1
17:30 Min	3½ MPH	1
20:00 Min	3 MPH	1

If you prefer, you can even use a motorized treadmill for taking the 12-minute fitness test, providing you have an accurate speedometer. Set the treadmill at the required speed for a given fitness category, then see if you can stay on the treadmill for 12 minutes. If so, you know that you meet the requirements for that particular fitness category. For example, the following chart provides guidelines for the 12-minute fitness test for men under 30 years of age.

REQUIREMENTS FOR 12-MINUTE FITNESS TEST ON
MOTORIZED TREADMILL

(for men under 30 years of age)

Treadmill Speed	Time Endured on Treadmill	Fitness Category
5 MPH	less than 12 Min	I. Very Poor
5–6 MPH	12:00 Min	II. Poor
6¼–7¼ MPH	12:00 Min	III. Fair
7½–9 MPH	12:00 Min	IV. Good
Over 9 MPH	12:00 Min	V. Excellent

There is no inherent advantage in taking a fitness test on

the treadmill instead of running out in the open. But it does eliminate such difficulties as finding a track, measuring off the distance you cover in 12 minutes, and worrying about what the neighbors will think when they see you huffing and puffing down the road.

In this chapter, I have discussed some of the devices that may be used in an indoor aerobics program, or to augment an outdoor program when weather conditions or other circumstances make outdoor exercise impractical. There are other kinds of indoor exercise machines, but the ones mentioned here are the most efficient and the easiest to use.

It has been my observation, however, that many people who purchase expensive exercise equipment use it for only a short time and then store it, evidently preferring outdoor exercise (or no exercise at all). That is why, at the conclusion of this chapter, I want to reemphasize what I have said many times before: to practice aerobics you really don't need equipment of any kind.

11: I'm Glad You Asked Me . . .

QUESTIONS AND ANSWERS are one of the best ways to clear up areas of confusion. That's why, after a lecture, I usually invite questions from the audience. It is encouraging to see how many excellent and thought provoking questions are asked during these discussion periods.

From the thousands of questions posed by my lecture audiences and correspondents, I have picked a typical sampling. Some of them touch on basic principles of aerobic exercise, others on specific exercise problems; many are concerned with the point value of certain activities, the effect of smoking and drinking on fitness, the special requirements for athletes, and a variety of personal situations.

Despite the often personal character of these questions, I feel that they are of general interest. After all, it is the personal experience with exercise that puts basic principles in sharper focus, linking theory and practice.

BASIC PRINCIPLES

Q. I am 45 years old and have been working my way through the running conditioning program. But after about 12 weeks I hit a snag and still can't manage to reach 30 points per week. What should I do?

A. If you find that you cannot reach the 30-point-per-week level within the 16-week conditioning period suggested in the chart, just repeat the weekly assignment at whatever level you *can* reach. If necessary, lengthen the distance and increase the time to build up your point total. Remember it is possible to reach 30 points per week just by walking.

Q. You say that the vast majority of your test subjects respond to the 30-point per week routine and easily meet the minimum test requirement. Why don't the others respond?

A. One always has to allow for individual differences. However, most of those who failed to respond were handicapped by heavy smoking, obesity, or both. Some quit smoking and reduced their weight. After that, even they responded to the 30-point regimen and showed improved aerobic capacity.

Q. My brother and I are having an argument. He says it's speed that really counts in earning your points. I say the most important thing is the distance you cover. Who's right?

A. Neither. Aerobic points are earned by a combination of both factors. Concentrate on earning points, and don't worry about setting speed or distance records. As a general rule I advise against striving for speed, which increases strain and fatigue. You can earn your points more safely and more comfortably by exercising at a slower rate for a longer time.

Q. After a game of handball, my pulse checks out around 160. That's what you say it should be. But I still don't understand what pulse rate means in term of aerobics.

A. Two factors are essential in producing the aerobic training effect. The exercise must be 1) strenuous enough, and 2) long enough. Your pulse shows that your handball game is certainly strenuous enough.

In the average person under 30 years of age, a heart rate of 150 beats per minute means that he is working at about 60 percent of his maximum capacity. For young, healthy people, that's a good energy level for producing a training effect.

However, the training effect can be reached in other ways: you may either work for a short time at a high heart rate or you may work for a longer time at a slower heart rate. The following chart, in simplified form, shows some of the possible combinations which can be used in producing a training effect.

Training Effect

Daily Time Requirements (Min)	180	90	45	20	10
Working Capacity (% of Maximum)	20	30	40	50	60
Heart Rate (beats per min)	110	120	130	140	150

The longer exercise periods are more realistic for older people whereas the exercise for younger people can be harder and shorter.

Q. I've been lifting weights for many years. After pushing up a heavy bar, I can feel my heart pounding very fast. Does this mean that I'm getting an aerobic effect?

A. Weight lifting is an isotonic exercise, and even though it accelerates the heart rate, it has little aerobic effect. If you just strain against the heavy weight, you tense your muscles, but there is no rapid movement. Such static exercise does not increase blood flow. The heart beats under the strain, but the static muscles return little blood to the heart. Therefore, the fast beat does not produce greater blood flow volume. This deprives the exercise of its aerobic value.

You'd be better off to use light weights and push them up and down rapidly to create continuous movement. Even so, it would require at least 30–45 minutes of activity to yield any appreciable number of aerobic points. Weight lifting is fine for muscle building. But remember that muscle size and strength are not always indicative of aerobic fitness.

Q. I'm with you when you say that exercise should be a family affair. Fortunately, my whole family is crazy about bowling. We've got a regular bowling date twice a week and spend about two hours at the alley. How do we figure points for that?

A. Sorry to disappoint you. I realize that bowling is great fun, but from an aerobic viewpoint, it's of little value. When you swing the ball, you're doing intense muscular work. But that lasts only a few seconds. Then you stand around again, waiting for the strike, waiting for the second ball, or just waiting your turn. Out of the whole game you only get very few minutes of actual muscular effort, and even that is not continuous. That's why I can't award points for bowling.

Q. One of my favorite summer recreations is skulling, and I keep in condition during the cold months with an indoor rowing machine. Can I earn my aerobic points that way?

A. Indeed you can, at the rate of 1 point for every six minutes if you row at a rate of 20 strokes per minute with both oars. Remember, though, that rowing does not involve the legs extensively. Therefore, you might supplement your rowing with running, cycling, walking, etc. Whenever the weather permits.

Q. I'm 56, and my doctor says aerobics is too tough for a man of my age. Walking 20 minutes twice a day, he says, is all the exercise I need. What do you think?

A. Ask your doctor to look up the charts. He'll find that covering 1.5 miles in 21:30 minutes earns 3 points. Twice a day, five times a week, this adds up to 30 points. So it seems that your doctor suggests exactly what I suggest. If he'd figure it out according to the charts, he may find that aerobics isn't "too tough" after all.

SMOKING AND DRINKING

A surprising number of questions come from people worried about the effect of smoking and drinking on their physical fitness. I had a feeling that some of my questioners were looking for reassurance, hoping I'd tell them that smoking and drinking don't really matter. My answers must have disappointed them.

Q. I have been smoking for 15 years. I try to hold it down to a pack a day, but I can't quit. I know I may get cancer, emphysema, bronchitis, and whatnot. But right now I'm basically healthy. I don't have any of these ailments. So how does smoking limit my physical performance?

A. An athlete I know was asked why he quit smoking. His simple, direct answer, based on his personal experience, sums up the problem: "It cuts your wind."

Behind this simple fact lie some grim medical details. You consider yourself "basically healthy." Frankly, I doubt that there is such a thing as a basically healthy smoker. Even if lung cancer and other smoking-related diseases have yet to catch up with you, you are partially disabled as soon as you smoke your first pack. According to information compiled by the American Medical Association, just ten puffs of a cigarette increase resistance in the air pathways of the lungs. This choked-up condition persists for an hour after each smoke.

Your physical performance is affected when you smoke because the body loses some of its ability to transport oxygen from the lungs to the muscles. Carbon monoxide in cigarette smoke is a potent poison that rapidly enters the blood, combines with the hemoglobin in the red blood corpuscles and renders many of them incapable of carrying oxygen.

The lung capacity of habitual smokers gradually shrinks, the membranes of their air passages thicken and become less efficient in gas exchange. Moreover, the cilia (tiny hairlike structures acting as brooms to sweep out the windpipe and the bronchial tubes) become paralyzed by cigarette smoking. Without this natural defense, the lungs are vulnerable to airborne intruders, dust particles and other pollutants.

The total picture is this: Smoking creates the opposite effect from aerobics. It wrecks the body's ability to absorb and distribute oxygen.

Q. How can I, as a compulsive smoker, benefit from aerobics?

A. Smoking has been called slow suicide. It may take longer to kill yourself if aerobics is able to counteract some of the damage from smoking.

Q. Like the guy in the joke, I quit smoking—twice a week. Each time I try, I backslide. Can aerobics do anything for someone like me?

A. If you have a sincere desire to quit, aerobic conditioning can help you break the habit. Several reformed smokers tell me that aerobics helped them get rid of their craving for tobacco.

We still don't know for sure why this is so. It may be that regular exercise gives you a sense of positive achievement that bolsters your willpower. Very likely, the physical changes resulting from exercise also play a role in curing the habit. This area has yet to be explored.

Q. Everybody says alcohol and athletics don't mix. I like to keep in shape, but I also like a drink before dinner—a small one. Will this interfere with my fitness training?

A. It depends on your individual reaction. Some people can tolerate small amounts of alcohol without impairing their physical performance. Others find it impossible to get anywhere near their top performance with any alcohol intake, no matter how small. That is why many professional athletes refrain from alcohol for at least 36 to 48 hours before a sports event.

Since individual tolerance varies so greatly, it is difficult to set standards other than to say that abstinence is the only absolute way to assure no impairment in performance.

MAINLY FOR ATHLETES

Those preparing for competitive sports approach aerobics with a point of view different from those interested mainly in personal fitness. Their questions reflect this difference.

Q. Everyone on our team is sold on aerobics, we play soccer—and that takes a lot of running and endurance. But the head of our physical education department still believes that calisthenics is better for athletic conditioning. So which is it—calisthenics or aerobics?

A. Many college, university and professional athletic teams have asked me this question. I usually suggest an aerobics program supplemented by short-distance sprinting and calisthenics. An athlete so trained gains a blend of speed, coordination and endurance that gives him an edge in almost any sport.

Q. As a college athlete (track and basketball), I'm interested in building up my staying power for competition. How many points per week do you recommend for this purpose?

A. For athletic conditioning I suggest at least 50 points per week off-season and at least 100 points per week during the season. Many athletes in training do considerably more, earning up to 300 and 400 points per week.

Q. I timed myself for a quarter mile. Sixty-three seconds! How does this rate for fitness?

A. It doesn't. You're fast all right. But dash speed (anaerobics) is unrelated to basic fitness, for short bursts of energy are not indicative of heart-lung reserve. What counts is endurance (aerobics) which is a direct measure of heart-lung capacity. Take the 12-minute test or the 1.5 mile test and find out how fit you really are.

Q. I'm a pretty fast runner and worked my way up into Category V. Now I'd like to find out how I stack up in competition with people of my age. I'm not in college and don't belong to any sports club. Where could I find out?

A. Your best bet is to check with the National Jogging Association, P.O. Box 19367, Washington, D.C. 20036; the Mile-a-Thon International, c/o Long Beach Community Hospital, 1720 Termino Avenue, Long Beach, California, 90804; Road Runners Club of America, 1584 Spruce Drive, Kalamazoo, Michigan, 49005 or your local "Y." Chances are that one of them would know about amateur sports competitions in your area. An increasing number of communities are now organizing public "Run-for-Fun" programs. Perhaps you can join one of those. The best known event open to male competitors of all ages is the Boston Marathon, an annual 26-

mile race from Hopkinton to Boston, Massachusetts. Last year, more than a thousand people came to Boston from all over the world to join in.

Q. I go out for track at my high school, so I'm naturally interested in speed. But the aerobic charts don't list point values for fast running—nothing at all for a guy who breaks 5:00 minutes for a mile. Why don't you figure out points for fellows who are really fast on their feet?

A. I have not measured oxygen consumption or assigned aerobic points in that speed range because I consider it of very limited applicability. The charts are intended primarily for fitness training rather than competitive sports. Besides, I don't encourage high speed as a goal in running exercise— at any rate not for the general public. Speed makes massive demands on the heart that may be dangerous to older or deconditioned persons. As a rule I favor earning points in a less strenuous manner by running at a slower rate for a longer distance.

Q. As a basketball player, I use aerobics to build up my endurance. Some weeks I earn as many as 200 points. But at the end of a workout I sometimes get a strange feeling in my chest. It's not a pain. It just feels hollow, as if there were an empty space around my heart. Is that normal?

A. That hollow feeling in your chest is probably a premature ventricular contraction (PVC). It's a kind of extra heartbeat sandwiched into the regular heart rhythm. This is fairly common among athletes engaged in strenuous exercise. It's not dangerous as such, but it may be a sign that you are driving yourself too hard, and there is always a certain risk in getting close to the limit of your capacity. I'd suggest that you reduce the intensity of your exercise but first, let your family doctor evaluate you.

Q. I saw a TV commercial in which professional athletes endorsed a vitamin product. They claim vitamin C and E improve their performance. What is your opinion?

A. As yet, it has not been conclusively demonstrated that vitamin supplements beyond the daily minimum requirement have any effect at all on athletic performance. At the Squadron Officers School, Maxwell Air Force Base, Alabama, a test of vitamin C involved 286 men engaged in a 12-week vigorous conditioning program. Half of the men received ten times the daily requirement; the other half re-

ceived no supplement to a normal diet. Everyone participated in games of flickerball, volleyball, and soccer and, in
addition, they were tested on the 12-minute endurance test
at the beginning and end of training. At the conclusion of
the study, the two groups revealed no significant difference
in athletic or endurance performance, the frequency of injuries, or the speed of recovery.

A similar research project on vitamin E is being contem-
plated, but so far the study has not been performed.

INDOOR EXERCISE

A surprising number of inquiries concern indoor exercise. Here are a few samples of more than routine interest.

Q. I exercise at home on a stationary bike. But mine
doesn't have a speedometer or mileage counter. This makes
it impossible for me to use the charts of the cycling program.
Can you give me some other guidelines?

A. It may be possible for you to have a speedometer/
odometer installed on your stationary bike. But if not, you
might try to do the following. Start with a 5:00 minute exercise period and add 1:00 minute per week until you work
up to 20:00 minutes per day, six days per week. Continue to
increase the brake resistance as your physical condition improves. Adjust the brake force so that at the end of each
exercise period you feel moderately fatigued but not un-
comfortably exhausted. By this I mean that your breathing
should be back to normal and your heart rate 100 or less ten
minutes after the exercise. If you cannot meet these requirements, adjust the bike for easier pedaling.

Q. I use a treadmill for indoor exercise, but I find that I
have to hold on to the rails to keep my balance. I realize
that grasping the rail lessens the aerobic effect. How many
points should I deduct? I usually walk an 18-minute mile
up a 15 percent incline.

A. Normally, an 18-minute mile on a self-propelled treadmill with a 15 percent incline is worth 3 points. Yet, it is
difficult to measure the energy requirement when holding
on to the rails. For this reason, I would encourage you to
learn to walk without holding on to the side rails but if
necessary hold on and subtract one point per mile.

Q. As a young girl I used to go to ballet class. Now that

I'm a middle-aged housewife, I still like to do an occasional pirouette in the living room. I wonder if dancing earns me any aerobic points?

A. It depends on what kind of dancing you do. Slow ballet movements in the style of the "Dying Swan" will do little to increase your aerobic capacity. By contrast, fast-moving ballet numbers, many kinds of modern dancing, and vigorous folk dances with fast footwork unquestionably have some aerobic effect. But because dances differ so greatly, it has not been possible to assign representative point values.

KEEPING SCORE

Questions about point credits are by far the most frequent. Some of these queries are about the charts themselves while others concern modes of exercise not specifically covered by the charts.

Q. One of the things I like about aerobics is that everything follows quite logically from a basic principle. But the logic of the point charts sometimes puzzles me. For example, you're giving me 5 points for running a mile in 6:30 minutes. And you're giving me 5 points for running a mile in 7:59 minutes. How come? Shouldn't I earn more points for running faster?

A. Of course you should. But I set up the charts so that the point credits increase in steps rather than as a continuous curve. Credit represents the slowest performance within each step. This is the reason for the apparent discrepancy.

Setting up the charts in this way allows a certain margin for error. It assures that you are getting all the exercise you need for effective conditioning even if there is a slight error in your measurement of time or distance.

Q. I get most of my walking exercise near my home in the Green Mountains of Vermont. A beautiful path near my house leads up to a fine lookout point. I go there almost every afternoon, and then back home again. Should I get extra credit because of the hilly terrain?

A. If the uphill and downhill parts of your course are approximately equal, the effect of incline cancels out and you get no extra points. But if you walked a course that is more uphill than downhill, you certainly should award yourself extra points.

You can figure the added points for various grades of climb from the Inclination Chart in Chapter Ten (Page 151). For example, walking at a speed of 3.4 mph (18:00 minutes per mile) is worth 1 point on a level grade. But if you walk at the same speed up a 15 percent grade, the point value jumps to 3.

Q. I earn about 50 points per week, cycling on New Jersey back roads on my English three-speed racer. Would I have to figure my credit in a different way if I used a ten-speed racing bike or a standard no-shift bike?

A. Experience has shown that the difference in energy expended on various types of bicycles is not great enough to require adjustment of the point chart. Since the chart is set up to allow a certain margin for error, you'll be getting the total point value from your exercise even if you ride a ten-speed racer.

Q. I'm a commuter and ride my bike to and from the railroad station, a distance of one mile. I do this every day. How many points do I get?

A. Riding a mile on a bike probably doesn't take you more than four minutes. That's not long enough to reach a steady state of energy expenditure. As a result, no aerobic training effect can take place and you earn no points. Remember that to gain aerobic benefits (and point credits) your exercise must be long enough and must challenge the heart and lungs to supply higher than ordinary amounts of oxygen.

Q. Ever since we read about aerobics, my husband and I go out regularly for an early evening run. It's doing wonders for our health as well as our disposition. But there's one problem. He's 6'1" and I'm 5'3". With my short legs, I have to take almost twice as many steps as he. So I feel I'm entitled to some extra points.

A. Sorry to disappoint you, but laboratory measurements say "no extra points." I know this sounds unfair, but the energy expenditure of tall and short people running on the treadmill has been measured, and there is no significant difference once you compensate for body weight. Only the very short ones—below five feet in height—have to work harder to keep up.

Q. Do I get more points for running three continuous

miles in 24 minutes than for three separate miles, each one in less than eight minutes?

A. The training effect is the same in both cases, so you get the same number of points. I realize that instinctively you may feel a continuous three-mile run would earn more aerobic benefit than three separate mile runs. But according to our current data, it just doesn't seem to work out that way.

Q. I've been doing yoga exercises for some time and find them wonderfully relaxing. I wonder if I can get any aerobic points that way?

A. I know of no aerobic benefit from standing on your head or other yoga-type exercises. Many people derive muscular relaxation and other benefits from such exercises, but so far there has been no indication that they have any aerobic value.

TEACHER'S SEMINAR

Q. As head of the physical education department of a Georgia high school, I wish I could provide an incentive for exercise. How do you motivate boys and girls from 12 to 14 who are too young to care much about fitness?

A. At that age, children can be readily motivated by competition. Unlike younger age groups, they are mature enough not to be damaged in their character development by the competitive element. I know of several schools awarding patches to students achieving 30 points per week, another patch for 50 points, and a special "Century Club" emblem for 100 points. Of course, it should be made clear to the students that the "Century Club" is not for everyone. Nobody needs to feel left out for not getting in. Such intense level of exercise is primarily for athletes developing their "staying power." But the entire student body—except for those medically screened out—should be motivated to go for the 30 and 50 point patches.

Grades are also a good motivator. I was recently told of a high school in California that awards grades to boys in physical education based on performance in a one-mile run. You can't earn an "A" unless you run a mile faster than six minutes, seven minutes is required for a B, eight minutes for a C and longer than eight minutes means a D. During a recent semester, 97 percent of the students got passing grades.

Q. I supervise physical education classes for children from seven to 14 years. Can you suggest types of exercise and aerobic goals for this age group?

A. Walking, running, cycling and swimming are excellent even for the younger children. The older children, from about ten years up, may take part in more competitive team sports. As yet, we do not have enough data to set aerobic norms for children in the six to ten age bracket. I assume that about 20 points per week would not be an unrealistic requirement. Above the age of ten, the weekly minimum is the same as for adults—30 points per week.

SPECIAL SITUATIONS

Q. I'm 55 years old and, try as I may, I can't meet the time goals in the chart. What do you advise?

A. You probably have been trying to meet the time goal in the original charts which did not provide for age adjustment. Instead, follow the age-adjusted chart in this book. You may find it much easier. Then, if you still have trouble meeting the specified time goals, exercise at a slower speed. That way you can still get your 30 points per week and remember that it is more important to get your points than it is to reach a specific time goal.

Q. Back in 1960 I had a slight myocardial infarction. In October I suffered another slight heart attack. With this history, do you think aerobics is safe for me?

A. Only your own doctor can tell you, because only he has detailed knowledge of your condition. However, the cardiac walking program outlined in the Chart Pack has proved successful in the rehabilitation of many people who have suffered heart attacks. The objective is to train yourself so that you gradually reach the point where you can comfortably walk a mile in less than 14:30 minutes. Then you work up to three miles a day, or 1½ miles twice a day, five days a week. This gives you 30 points per week, which gives you enough of an aerobic training effect to build up your cardiovascular reserve. It may take you 32 weeks or even longer to reach this point. Do not rush it. And do not even start any exercise program without the specific approval of your physician.

Q. My pulse rate at rest is between 48 and 52—about six beats per minute slower than when I started the aerobics program about four months ago. But I notice that it takes nearly an hour for my heart rate to return to normal after I run an eight-minute mile. After a two-mile run it takes even longer. Is that okay?

A. It's all right as long as your heart rate returns to about 100 after ten minutes of rest. To drop back to the normal resting rate may take a good deal longer. What happens is this: The oxygen debt you build up during aerobic exercise is mostly "paid back" during the first few minutes after exercise, and your heartbeat slows considerably during that period. But to pay back the rest of the accumulated oxygen debt may take as long as one to three hours, depending on how hard you exercised. As long as you are repaying, your heart must pump more than the normal amount of blood. Hence your heart rate will remain slightly elevated.

Q. An old knee injury prevents me from running, and even walking isn't comfortable. Yet with my 215 pounds and 48 years, I definitely need exercise. My doctor suggests swimming, since that would put the least strain on my knee. The problem is that I can't afford a swimming pool. Any other suggestions?

A. I realize that a standard-size, concrete swimming pool would be expensive, but you might consider one of those inexpensive round plastic pools that are entirely above ground and can be easily put up in the yard. Then get a swimming harness and tether it to the rim of the pool. That way you can "swim in place" in a small pool.

One man I know exercises in this way, using the time chart for the swimming program. Of course he can't gauge his "distance" while swimming on a tether. Instead, he checks his pulse after the specified time period, making sure he is swimming fast enough to drive his heart rate to 140. Occasionaly he swims at a friend's regular pool where he can measure his distance. This gives him a chance to check his performance directly against the chart.

Another possibility you and your doctor might consider is an indoor rowing machine. Many people handicapped in the use of their legs have found such machines a suitable exercise device. The seat could be screwed down in a fixed position so that no flexing of the knees occurs.

Q. Sunday is my only chance to get in a few sets of tennis. Frankly, I think a once-a-week workout is better than nothing at all. Why then are you so hard on us "weekend athletes"?

A. Your motives are fine, but your methods are something else again. For one thing, Sunday-only exercise gives you very little aerobic benefit. The intervening week is too long an interruption. No significant training effect can possibly occur. Worse yet, weekend athletes are a danger to themselves. The sudden Sunday exertion can be harmful unless you are conditioned by regular weekday exercise.

Q. I'm about 20 pounds too heavy and have been trying to shake off some of that extra fat by running. How many calories can I burn up that way?

A. Figure about 100 calories for an eight-minute mile. That's not enough to whittle down that extra weight of yours rapidly. You'd have to run three miles a day to burn enough calories to obtain a significant weight reduction. But if you supplement your running with a moderate diet, even one mile a day will soon give you results.

Q. How can I tell if I push myself too hard during the conditioning period?

A. Fatigue is a good general indicator. If you feel tired most of the time—not just for an hour or so after exercising —you are probably driving yourself too hard. More specifically, you can check your recovery heart rate. As I have mentioned before, five minutes after exercise your heart rate should be less than 120, ten minutes after exercise it should be less than 100. If your heart rate at those time points is faster than that, cut back on your exercise.

Q. I've just an ordinary cold. Should I continue to exercise? I hate to miss out on my conditioning program.

A. You should never exercise while you suffer from an acute infection—and a common cold is just that. Also stop exercising if you have the flu, an intestinal upset or other virus disorders. If you have a fever, wait until your temperature returns to normal. Then wait at least an additional 24 hours. Not before then should you resume exercise—and then at a slower pace than before your illness.

Q. I never had any trouble with brittle bones before, but after five weeks of running on the aerobics program, I cracked a bone in my left foot. It's six weeks later now and it no longer hurts. Can I go back to the conditioning program now?

A. Better wait a while yet. It is important to give a fracture enough time to heal completely before putting renewed stress on it. Absence of pain is a sign that the fracture is at least partially healed, but your doctor should make the final decision about your reentry into the conditioning program.

It may interest you to know that frequently a bone becomes stronger after a break. The strengthening effect results from the thickening of the bone at the point of fracture and from drawing more calcium into the tissue during the healing process.

When your doctor says you can resume exercise, don't start running right away. Stick with the walking program for a few weeks. If no complications occur, you may then switch to running again.

Q. About six weeks after I started on the running program, I began to feel stiff around neck and shoulders. What do you think is the reason?

A. Very likely you are not using your arms properly while running. Chances are that you are tense and carry your arms far too high. Relax and let your arms swing loose as you run. The natural rhythm of their swing will add to your forward momentum, making your overall body movement more efficient. Also, you may benefit from some calisthenic exercises for the arms.

Q. Sometimes I feel quite giddy during or after exercise, sort of light-headed and dizzy. Is that normal?

A. Your symptom is not normal. It may be due to hyperventilation, which means that you're breathing in and out more than you need to. That way you blow off carbon dioxide, changing the chemical balance of the blood. This, in turn, affects the brain and makes you dizzy.

It is also possible that your dizziness is caused by insufficient blood supply to the brain due to a heart or blood vessel problem. In that case you should not be exercising at all. So let your doctor check you out, just to be sure.

Q. Should I exercise when I'm fatigued from overwork or lack of sleep?

A. No, skip exercising that day. Unusual fatigue, inadequate sleep or excessive emotional strain, added to vigorous exercise, may cause undesirable consequences.

I would like to finish up this chapter with one of the toughest questions I ever fielded from the lecture platform. I was speaking in Oklahoma City, Oklahoma, when a large man rose in the audience and said: "I've been trying to explain aerobics to my wife. But the more I try, the more I get mixed up. Finally she asked me, 'Can you define aerobics in a single sentence?' So that's what I'm asking you."

Being accustomed to talking for hours on aerobics, I must admit that momentarily I was stumped. But then I made a brave try at a simple answer: "Aerobics is a system of exercise designed to improve your overall health, but particularly the condition of the heart, lungs and blood vessels." This doesn't tell all, of course, but it does sum it up.

An Afterthought

IN THE RELATIVELY short span of fifty years, the automobile has so altered our way of life that walking—the most natural mode of locomotion—now seems almost discreditable.

I once expressed this thought to a friend who is a successful car dealer.

Predictably, he responded.

"I hate to see cars getting the blame for everything," he said irritabily. "I bet people didn't walk any more in the old days than they do now. They just went by horse and buggy."

"When you went to school," I asked, "how did you get there?"

He admitted that he had walked more than three miles to and from school.

"And your children?"

"The bus picks them up."

"And does your wife use a car much?"

"Oh yes, you should see our monthly gasoline bill."

I didn't press my point further.

No, the automobile is not just a mechanical replacement for the horse. It represents an entirely new attitude, a new set of customs, and it is ushering in an era of physical passivity.

I remember when people walked to church, to the store and the post office. Today, we have the "drive-in craze." There are drive-in restaurants, drive-in cleaners, drive-in theaters and drive-in banks. Not only have we given up walking; we don't even get out of the car when we reach our destinations!

Paradoxically, this passion for passivity extends even to sports, robbing them of much of their healthful effects. The golf cart and the ski lift are but two of many examples of our unwillingness or inability to move under our own power. And we are becoming so engrossed with television that a major portion of our leisure time, formerly spent in outdoor activities, is now spent in watching television. To top that, remote control is making it "out of style" to leave the comfortable, cushioned chair to change television stations. Where will it end?

But all of these changes have been too swift for the human organism. Over many thousands of years, since before the dawn of civilization, our bodies have been geared to and sustained by habitual and extensive physical activity. Now, with dramatic suddenness, this functional pattern has been broken. Our legs are technologically unemployed. And our entire health suffers for it.

Even in other areas of our modern life, strenuous physical activity is a thing of the past. Mechanization has placed the farmer in the driver's seat, the construction worker at the controls of a crane, and the road builder on his bulldozer. The warehouseman has his fork lifts, the carpenter his power tools, and the office-worker his elevators to eliminate the occasional effort of climbing a flight of stairs. Even the trucker—thanks to power steering and power brakes—exerts little more muscular effort than the housewife driving to a bridge party.

Unquestionably, these developments represent progress. Modern technology has created immense benefits and satisfied many human needs. I am not criticizing these accomplishments, and I am certainly not suggesting that we tear up our highways, junk our cars, and eliminate the elevators. But, as a physician, I am concerned about the medical consequences of the machine age. The high tension and low activity of modern life make a deadly mixture. Biologically, we're in the midst of a crisis, and the statistics on cardiovascular disease show it.

At this point in the history of civilization, it is evident that technical progress may backfire unless it is matched by a balancing regard for human health and well-being. In its broadest sense, the question is whether man can prosper in the technological environment he has created. He must learn to protect the natural resources that sustain his life. He must learn to clean up the air and the water, and to preserve the land. But first of all, he must protect his own body against the ravages imposed by modern life.

It is my hope that aerobics will help him do so.

Appendix: The Point System Expanded. With the Addition of Endurance Points

1. WALKING/RUNNING

(at 1/10-Mile Increments)

In measuring a course that starts and finishes in front of their home, many people have found that it is impossible to end on an even mile or half-mile. Consequently, hundreds have asked for a chart that gives the point value for walking and running distances measured in 1/10 miles. The following special chart is in response to this request and gives the point value for walking and running one to five miles at 1/10-mile increments.

1.0 Mile

19:59—14:30 min	1
14:29—12:00 min	2
11:59—10:00 min	3
9:59— 8:00 min	4
7:59— 6:31 min	5
6:30— 5:45 min	6
under 5:45 min	7

1.1 Miles

21:59—15:57 min	1⅛
15:56—13:12 min	2¼
13:11—11:00 min	3⅓
10:59— 8:48 min	4½
8:47— 7:09 min	5½
7:08— 6:20 min	6⅔
under 6:20 min	7¾

1.2 Miles

23:59—17:24 min	1¼
17:23—14:24 min	2½
14:23—12:00 min	3⅔
11:59— 9:36 min	5
9:35— 7:48 min	6
7:47— 6.55 min	7⅓
under 6:55 min	8½

1.3 Miles

25:59—18:51 min	1⅜
18:50—15:36 min	2¾
15:35—13:00 min	4
12:59—10:24 min	5½

1.3 Miles (Cont.)

10:23— 8:27 min	6½
8:26— 7:30 min	8
under 7:30 min	9¼

1.4 Miles

27:59—20:18 min	1½
20:17—16:48 min	2¾
16:47—14:00 min	4½
13:59—11:00 min	6
10:59— 9:06 min	7
9:05— 8:05 min	8⅔
under 8:05 min	10

1.5 Miles

29:59—21:45 min	1½
21:44—18:00 min	3
17:59—15:00 min	4½
14:59—12:00 min	6
11:59— 9:45 min	7½
9:44— 8:40 min	9
under 8:40 min	10½

1.6 Miles

31:59—23:12 min	1⅝
23:11—19:12 min	3¼
19:11—16:00 min	4⅔
15:59—12:48 min	6½
12:47—10:24 min	8
10:23— 9:15 min	9⅔
under 9:15 min	11¼

1. WALKING/RUNNING (CONTINUED)
(at 1/10-Mile Increments)

1.7 Miles

33:59—24:39 min	1¾
24:38—20:24 min	3½
20:23—17:00 min	5
16:59—13:36 min	7
13:35—11:03 min	8½
11:02— 9:50 min	10⅓
under 9:50 min	12

1.8 Miles

35:59—26:06 min	1⅞
26:05—21:36 min	3¾
21:35—18:00 min	5⅓
17:59—14:24 min	7½
14:23—11:42 min	9
11:41—10:25 min	11
under 10:25 min	12¾

1.9 Miles

37:59—27:33 min	1⅞
27:32—22:48 min	3¾
22:47—19:00 min	5⅔
18:59—15:12 min	7½
15:11—12:21 min	9½
12:20—11:00 min	11½
under 11:00 min	13½

2.0 Miles

40:00 min or longer	1*
39:59—29:00 min	2
28:59—24:00 min	4
23:59—20:00 min	7
19:59—16:00 min	9
15:59—13:00 min	11
12:59—11:30 min	13
under 11:30 min	15

2.1 Miles

42:00 min or longer	1*
41:59—30:27 min	2⅛
30:26—25:12 min	4¼
25:11—21:00 min	7½

2.1 Miles (Cont.)

20:59—16:48 min	9⅔
16:47—13:39 min	11¾
13:38—12:05 min	13¾
under 12:05 min	16

2.2 Miles

44:00 min or longer	1*
43:59—31:54 min	2¼
31:53—26:24 min	4½
26:23—22:00 min	7¾
21:59—17:36 min	10
17:35—14:18 min	12¼
14:17—12:40 min	14½
under 12:40 min	16⅔

2.3 Miles

46:00 min or longer	1*
45:59—33:21 min	2⅜
33:20—27:36 min	4¾
27:35—23:00 min	8⅓
22:59—18:24 min	10⅔
18:23—14:57 min	13
14:56—13:15 min	15⅓
under 13:15 min	17⅔

2.4 Miles

48:00 min or longer	1*
47:59—34:48 min	2½
34:47—28:48 min	4¾
28:47—24:00 min	8⅔
23:59—19:12 min	11
19:11—15:36 min	13½
15:35—13:50 min	16
under 13:50 min	18¼

2.5 Miles

50:00 min or longer	1*
49:59—36:15 min	2½
36:14—30:00 min	5
29:59—25:00 min	9
24:59—20:00 min	11½
19:59—16:15 min	14

* Exercise of sufficient duration to be of cardiovascular benefit. At this speed, ordinarily no training effect would occur. However, the duration is of such extent that a training effect does begin to occur.

1. WALKING/RUNNING (CONTINUED)
(at 1/10-Mile Increments)

2.5 Miles (Cont.)

16:14—14:20 min	16½
under 14:20 min	19

2.6 Miles

52:00 min or longer	1*
51:59—37:42 min	2⅝
37:41—31:12 min	5¼
31:11—26:00 min	9¼
25:59—20:48 min	12
20:47—16:54 min	14½
16:53—15:00 min	17
under 15:00 min	19½

2.7 Miles

54:00 min or longer	1*
53:59—39:09 min	2¾
39:08—32:24 min	5½
32:23—27:00 min	9½
26:59—21:36 min	12½
21:35—17:33 min	15
17:32—15:35 min	18
under 15:35 min	20¼

2.8 Miles

56:00 min or longer	1*
55:59—40:36 min	2⅞
40:35—33:36 min	5¾
33:35—28:00 min	10
27:59—22:24 min	13
22:23—18:12 min	15½
18:11—16:10 min	18½
under 16:10 min	21

2.9 Miles

58:00 min or longer	1*
57:59—42:03 min	2⅞
42:01—34:48 min	5¾
34:47—29:00 min	10½
28:59—23:12 min	13¼
23:11—18:51 min	16¼
18:50—16:45 min	19
under 16:45 min	22

3.0 Miles

1 hr or longer	1½*
59:59—43:30 min	3
43:29—36:00 min	6
35:59—30:00 min	11
29:59—24:00 min	14
23:59—19:30 min	17
19:29—17:15 min	20
under 17:15 min	23

3.1 Miles

1 hr 2:00 min or longer	1½*
1 hr 1:59—44:57 min	3⅛
44:56—37:12 min	6¼
37:11—31:00 min	11½
30:59—24:48 min	14½
24:47—20:10 min	17¾
20:09—17:50 min	20¾
under 17:50 min	24

3.2 Miles

1 hr 4:00 min or longer	1½*
1 hr 3:59—46:24 min	3¼
46:23—38:24 min	6½
38:23—32:00 min	11¾
31:59—25:36 min	15
25:35—20:49 min	18½
20:48—18:25 min	21¾
under 18:25 min	24⅔

3.3 Miles

1 hr 6 min or longer	1½*
1 hr 5:59—47:51 min	3⅜
47:50—39:36 min	6¾
39:35—33:00 min	12
32:59—26:24 min	15½
26:23—21:28 min	19
21:27—19:00 min	22½
under 19:00 min	25⅓

3.4 Miles

1 hr 8:00 min or longer	1½*
1 hr 7:59—49:18 min	3⅜

* Exercise of sufficient duration to be of cardiovascular benefit. At this speed, ordinarily no training effect would occur. However, the duration is of such extent that a training effect does begin to occur.

1. WALKING/RUNNING (CONTINUED)
(at 1/10-Mile Increments)

3.4 Miles (Cont.)

49:17—40:48 min	6¾
40:47—34:00 min	12½
33:59—27:12 min	16
27:11—22:07 min	19½
22:06—19:35 min	23
under 19:35 min	26

3.5 Miles

1 hr 10:00 min or longer	1½*
1 hr 9:59—50:45 min	3½
50:44—42:00 min	7
41:59—35:00 min	13
34:59—28:00 min	16½
27:59—22:45 min	20
22:44—20:10 min	23½
under 20:10 min	27

3.6 Miles

1 hr 12:00 min or longer	1½*
1 hr 11:59—52:12 min	3⅝
52:11—43:12 min	7¼
43:11—36:00 min	13½
35:59—28:48 min	17
28:47—23:24 min	20½
23:23—20:45 min	24¼
under 20:45 min	27¾

3.7 Miles

1 hr 14:00 min or longer	1½*
1 hr 13:59—53:39 min	3¾
53:38—44:24 min	7½
44:23—37:00 min	14
36:59—29:36 min	17½
29:35—24:03 min	21
24:02—21:15 min	25
under 21:15 min	28½

3.8 Miles

1 hr 16:00 min or longer	1½*
1 hr 15:59—55:06 min	3⅞
55:05—45:36 min	7¾
45:35—38:00 min	14

3.8 Miles (Cont.)

37:59—30:24 min	18
30:23—24:42 min	21¾
24:41—21:50 min	25¾
under 21:50 min	29¼

3.9 Miles

1 hr 18:00 min or longer	1½*
1 hr 17:59—56:33 min	3⅞
56:32—46:48 min	7¾
46:47—39:00 min	14½
38:59—31:12 min	18½
31:11—25:21 min	22½
25:20—22:25 min	26¼
under 22:25 min	30

4.0 Miles

1 hr 20:00 min or longer	4*
1 hr 19:59—58:00 min	7
57:59—48:00 min	11
47:59—40:00 min	15
39:59—32:00 min	19
31:59—26:00 min	23
25:59—23:00 min	27
under 23:00 min	31

4.1 Miles

1 hr 22:00 min or longer	4*
1 hr 21:59—59:27 min	7
59:26—49:12 min	11¼
49:11—41:00 min	15⅓
40:59—32:48 min	19½
32:47—26:39 min	23½
26:38—23:35 min	27½
under 23:35 min	31¾

4.2 Miles

1 hr 24:00 min or longer	4*
1 hr 23:59—60:54 min	7¼
60:53—50:24 min	11½
50:23—42:00 min	15⅔
41:59—33:36 min	20
33:35—27:18 min	24

* Exercise of sufficient duration to be of cardiovascular benefit. At this speed, ordinarily no training effect would occur. However, the duration is of such extent that a training effect does begin to occur.

1. WALKING/RUNNING (CONTINUED)
(at 1/10-Mile Increments)

4.2 Miles (Cont.)

27:17—24:10 min	28
under 24:10 min	32½

4.3 Miles

1 hr 26:00 min or longer	4*
1 hr 25:59—1 hr 2:21 min	7½
1 hr 2:20—51:36 min	11¾
51:35—43:00 min	16
42:59—34:24 min	20½
34:23—27:57 min	24½
27:56—24:45 min	28¾
under 24:45 min	33¼

4.4 Miles

1 hr 28:00 min or longer	4*
1 hr 27:59—1 hr 3:48 min	7¾
1 hr 3:47—52:48 min	12
52:47—44:00 min	16½
43:59—35:12 min	21
35:11—28:36 min	25¼
28:35—25:20 min	29½
under 25:20 min	34

4.5 Miles

1 hr 30:00 min or longer	4½*
1 hr 29:59—1 hr 5:15 min	8
1 hr 5:14—54:00 min	12½
53:59—45:00 min	17
44:59—36:00 min	21½
35:59—29:15 min	26
29:14—25:55 min	30½
under 25:55 min	35

4.6 Miles

1 hr 32:00 min or longer	4½*
1 hr 31:59—1 hr 6:42 min	8¼
1 hr 6:41—55:12 min	12¾
55:11—46:00 min	17½
45:59—36:48 min	22
36:47—29:54 min	26½
29:53—26:30 min	31
under 26:30 min	36

4.7 Miles

1 hr 34:00 min or longer	4½*
1 hr 33:59—1 hr 8:09 min	8¼
1 hr 8:08—56:24 min	13
56:23—47:00 min	18
46:59—37:36 min	22½
37:35—30:33 min	27
30:32—27:00 min	31½
under 27:00 min	37

4.8 Miles

1 hr 36:00 min or longer	4½*
1 hr 35:59—1 hr 9:36	8½
1 hr 9:35—57:36 min	13¼
57:35—48:00 min	18
47:59—38:24 min	23
38:23—31:12 min	27½
31:11—27:35 min	32
under 27:35 min	38

4.9 Miles

1 hr 38:00 min or longer	4½*
1 hr 37:59—1 hr 11:03 min	8¾
1 hr 11:02—58:48 min	13½
58:47—49:00 min	18½
48:59—39:12 min	23½
39:11—31:51 min	27½
31:50—28:10 min	33
under 28:10 min	38

5.0 Miles

1 hr 40:00 min or longer	5*
1 hr 39:59—1 hr 12:30 min	9
1 hr 12:29—1 hr	14
59:59—50:00 min	19
49:59—40:00 min	24
39:59—32:30 min	29
32:29—28:45 min	34
under 28:45 min	39

* Exercise of sufficient duration to be of cardiovascular benefit. At this speed, ordinarily no training effect would occur. However, the duration is of such extent that a training effect does begin to occur.

1. WALKING/RUNNING (CONTINUED)
(at 1/2-Mile Increments)

5.5 Miles

1 hr 50:00 min or longer	5½*
1 hr 49:59—1 hr 19:45 min	10
1 hr 19:44—1 hr 6:00 min	15½
1 hr 5:59—55:00 min	21
54:59—44:00 min	26½
43:59—35:45 min	32
35:44—31:35 min	37½
under 31:35 min	43

6.0 Miles

2 hrs or longer	6*
1 hr 59:59—1 hr 27:00 min	11
1 hr. 26:59—1 hr 12:00 min	17
1 hr 11:59—1 hr	23
59:59—48:00 min	29
47:59—39:00 min	35
38:59—34:30 min	41
under 34:30 min	47

6.5 Miles

2 hrs 10:00 min or longer	6½*
2 hrs 9:59—1 hr 34:15 min	12
1 hr 34:14—1 hr 18:00 min	18½
1 hr 17:59—1 hr 5:00 min	26
1 hr 4:59—52:00 min	32½
51:59—42:15 min	39
42:14—37:22 min	45½
under 37:22 min	52

7.0 Miles

2 hrs 20:00 min or longer	7*
2 hrs 19:59—1 hr 41:30 min	13
1 hr 41:29—1 hr 24:00 min	20
1 hr 23:59—1 hr 10:00 min	27
1 hr 9:59—56:00 min	34
55:59—45:30 min	41
45:29—40:15 min	48
under 40:15 min	55

7.5 Miles

2 hrs 30:00 min or longer	7½*
2 hrs 29:59—1 hr 48:45 min	14
1 hr 48:44—1 hr 30:00 min	21½
1 hr 29:59—1 hr 15:00 min	29
1 hr 14:59—60:00 min	36½
59:59—48:45 min	44
48:44—43:10 min	51½
under 43:10 min	59

8.0 Miles

2 hrs 40:00 min or longer	8*
2 hrs 39:59—1 hr 56:00 min	15
1 hr 55:59—1 hr 36:00 min	23
1 hr 35:59—1 hr 20:00 min	31
1 hr 19:59—1hr 4:00 min	39
1 hr 3:59—52:00 min	47
51:59—46:00 min	55
under 46:00 min	63

8.5 Miles

2 hrs 50:00 min or longer	8½*
2 hrs 49:59—2 hrs 3:15 min	16
2 hrs 3:14—1 hr 42:00 min	24½
1 hr 41:59—1 hr 25:00 min	33
1 hr 24:59—1 hr 8:00 min	41½
1 hr 7:59—55:15 min	50
55:14—48:50 min	58½
under 48:50 min	67

9.0 Miles

3 hrs or longer	9*
2 hrs 59:59—2 hrs 10:30 min	17
2 hrs 10:29—1 hr 48:00 min	26
1 hr 47:59—1 hr 30.00 min	35
1 hr 29:59—1 hr 12:00 min	44
1 hr 11:59—58:30 min	53
58:29—51:45 min	62
under 51:45 min	71

* Exercise of sufficient duration to be of cardiovascular benefit. At this speed, ordinarily no training effect would occur. However, the duration is of such extent that a training effect does begin to occur.

1. WALKING/RUNNING (CONTINUED)

9.5 Miles

3 hrs 10:00 min or longer	9*
3 hrs 9:59—2 hrs 17:45 min	18
2 hrs 17:44—1 hr 54:00 min	27½
1 hr 53:59—1 hr 35:00 min	37
1 hr 34:59—1 hr 16:00 min	46½
1 hr 15:59—1 hr 1:45 min	56
1 hr 1:44—54:40 min	65½
under 54:40 min	75

10.0 Miles

3 hrs 20:00 min or longer	10*
3 hrs 19:59—2 hrs 25:00 min	19
2 hrs 24:59—2 hrs	29
1 hr 59:59—1 hr 40:00 min	39
1 hr 39:59—1 hr 20:00 min	49
1 hr 19:59—1 hr 5:00 min	59
1 hr 4:59—57:30 min	69
under 57:30 min	79

12:5 Miles

3 hrs 1:15—2 hrs 30:00 min	36½
2 hrs 29:59—2 hrs 5:00 min	49
2 hrs 4:59—1 hr 40:00 min	61½
1 hr 39:59—1 hr 21:15 min	74
under 1 hr 21:15 min	86½

15 Miles

3 hrs 37:28 min—3 hrs	44
2 hrs 59:59—2 hrs 30:00 min	59
2 hrs 29:59—2 hrs	74
1 hr 59:59—1 hr 37:30 min	89
under 1 hr 37:30 min	104

20.0 Miles

4 hrs 49:59 min—4 hrs	59
3 hrs 59:59—3 hrs 20:00 min	79
3 hrs 19:59—2 hrs 40:00 min	99
2 hrs 39:59—2 hrs 10:00 min	119
under 22 hrs 10:00 min	139

25.0 Miles

6 hrs 2:25 min—5 hrs	74
4 hrs 59:59—4 hrs 10:00 min	99
4 hrs 9:59—3 hrs 20:00 min	124
3 hrs 19:59—2 hrs 42:30 min	149
under 2 hrs 42:30 min	174

MARATHON (26 Miles, 385 Yards)

Less than 2 hrs 30 min 45 sec	209
2 hrs 30:45—2 hrs 50:25 min	182
2 hrs 50:26—3 hrs 29:45 min	156
3 hrs 29:46—4 hrs 22:12 min	130
4 hrs 22:13—5 hrs 14:40 min	104
5 hrs 14:41—6 hrs 20:12 min	78
6 hrs 20:13—8 hrs 40:25 min	51

* Exercise of sufficient duration to be of cardiovascular benefit. At this speed, ordinarily no training effect would occur. However, the duration is of such extent that a training effect does begin to occur.

2. CYCLING

INSTRUCTIONS:

1. Points determined considering equal uphill and downhill course.
2. Points determined considering equal time with and against the wind.
3. For cycling a one-way course constantly against a wind exceeding 5 mph, add ½ point per mile to the total point value.

2.0 Miles

12 min or longer	0
11:59— 8:00 min	1
7:59— 6:00 min	2
under 6:00 min	3

3.0 Miles

18 min or longer	0
17:59—12:00 min	1½
11:59— 9:00 min	3
under 9:00 min	4½

4.0 Miles

24 min or longer	0
23:59—16:00 min	2
15:59—12:00 min	4
under 12:00 min	6

5.0 Miles

30 min or longer	1*
29:59—20:00 min	2½
19:59—15:00 min	5
under 15:00 min	7½

6.0 Miles

36 min or longer	1*
35:59—24:00 min	3
23:59—18:00 min	6
under 18:00 min	9

7.0 Miles

42 min or longer	3½*
41:59—28:00 min	5½
27:59—21:00 min	9
under 21:00 min	12½

8.0 Miles

48 min or longer	3½*
47:59—32:00 min	6½
31:59—24:00 min	10½
under 24:00 min	14½

9.0 Miles

54 min or longer	5*
53:59—36:00 min	7½
35:59—27:00 min	12
under 27:00 min	16½

10.0 Miles

1 hr or longer	5½*
59:59—40:00 min	8½
39:59—30:00 min	13½
under 30:00 min	18½

11.0 Miles

1 hr 6 min or longer	6½*
1 hr 5:59 min—44:00 min	9½
43:59—33:00 min	15
under 33:00 min	20½

12.0 Miles

1 hr 12 min or longer	7*
1 hr 11:59 min—48:00 min	10½
47:59—36:00 min	16½
under 36:00 min	22½

13.0 Miles

1 hr 18 min or longer	8*
1 hr 17:59 min—52:00 min	11½
51:59—39:00 min	18
under 39:00 min	24½

* Exercise of sufficient duration to be of cardiovascular benefit. At this speed, ordinarily no training effect would occur. However, the duration is of such extent that a training effect does begin to occur.

2. CYCLING (CONTINUED)

14.0 Miles

1 hr 24 min or longer	8½*
1 hr 23:59 min—56:00 min	12½
55:59—42:00 min	19½
under 42:00 min	26½

15.0 Miles

1 hr 30 min or longer	9½*
1 hr 29:59 min—1 hr	13½
59:59—45:00 min	21
under 45:00 min	28½

16.0 Miles

1 hr 36 min or longer	10*
1 hr 35:59 min—1 hr 4:00 min	14½
1 hr 3:59 min—48:00 min	22½
under 48:00 min	30½

17.0 Miles

1 hr 42:00 min or longer	11*
1 hr 41:50 min—1 hr 8 min	15½
1 hr 7:59 min—51:00 min	24
under 51:00 min	32½

18.0 Miles

1 hr 48:00 min or longer	11½*
1 hr 47:59 min—1 hr 12 min	16½
1 hr 11:59 min—54:00 min	25½
under 54:00 min	34½

19.0 Miles

1 hr 54:00 min or longer	12½
1 hr 53:59 min—1 hr 16 min	17½
1 hr 15:59 min—57:00 min	27
under 57:00 min	36½

20.0 Miles

2 hrs or longer	13*
1 hr 59:59 min—1 hr 20 min	18½
1 hr 19:59 min—1 hr	28½
under 1 hr	38½

25.0 Miles

2 hrs 30:00 min or longer	17*
2 hrs 29:59 min—1 hr 40 min	23½
1 hr 39:59 min—1 hr 15 min	36
under 1 hr 15:00 min	48½

30.0 Miles

3 hrs or longer	20½*
2 hrs 59:59 min—2 hrs	28½
1 hr 59:59 min—1 hr 30 min	43½
under 1 hr 30:00 min	58½

* Exercise of sufficient duration to be of cardiovascular benefit. At this speed, ordinarily no training effect would occur. However, the duration is of such extent that a training effect does begin to occur.

3. SWIMMING

200 Yards

6:40 min or longer	0
6:39— 5:00 min	1
4:59— 3:20 min	1½
under 3:20 min	2½

250 Yards

8:20 min or longer	0
8:19— 6:15 min	1¼
6:14— 4:10 min	2
under 4:10 min	3

300 Yards

10:00 min or longer	1*
9:59— 7:30 min	1½
7:29— 5:00 min	2½
under 5:00 min	3½

350 Yards

11:40 min or longer	1*
11:39— 8:45 min	2
8:44— 5:50 min	3
under 5:50 min	4½

400 Yards

13:20 min or longer	1*
13:19—10:00 min	2½
9:59— 6:40 min	3½
under 6:40 min	5

450 Yards

15:00 min or longer	1*
14:59—11:15 min	3
11:14— 7:30 min	4
under 7:30 min	5½

500 Yards

16:40 min or longer	1*
16:39—12:30 min	3
12:29— 8:20 min	4
under 8:20 min	6

550 Yards

18:20 min or longer	1*
18:19—13:45 min	3½
13:44— 9:10 min	4½
under 9:10 min	7

600 Yards

20:00 min or longer	1½*
19:59—15:00 min	4
14:59—10:00 min	5
under 10:00 min	7½

650 Yards

21:40 min or longer	1½*
21:39—16:15 min	4
16:14—10:50 min	5½
under 10:50 min	8

700 Yards

23:20 min or longer	1½*
23:19—17:30 min	4½
17:29—11:40 min	6
under 11:40 min	8½

750 Yards

25:00 min or longer	1½*
24:59—18:45 min	4¾
18:44—12:30 min	6½
under 12:30 min	9½

800 Yards

26:40 min or longer	2¼*
26:39—20:00 min	5¾
19:59—13:20 min	7¼
under 13:20 min	10¾

850 Yards

28:20 min or longer	2½*
28:19—21:15 min	6¼
21:14—14:10 min	8
under 14:10 min	11½

* Exercise of sufficient duration to be of cardiovascular benefit. At this speed, ordinarily no training effect would occur. However, the duration is of such extent that a training effect does begin to occur.

3. SWIMMING (CONTINUED)

900 Yards

30:00 min or longer	3¼*
29:59—22:30 min	6¾
22:29—15:00 min	8¾
under 15:00 min	12½

950 Yards

31:40 min or longer	3½*
31:39—23:15 min	7¼
23:14—15:50 min	9½
under 15:50 min	13½

1000 Yards

33:20 min or longer	4*
33:19—25:00 min	8¼
24:59—16:40 min	10½
under 16:40 min	14½

1100 Yards

36:40 min or longer	4½*
36:39—27:30 min	9½
27:29—18:20 min	11½
under 18:20 min	16¼

1200 Yards

40:00 min or longer	5½*
39:59—30:00 min	10½
29:59—20:00 min	13
under 20:00 min	18

1300 Yards

43:20 min or longer	6*
43:19—32:30 min	11½
32:29—21:40 min	14½
under 21:40 min	19¾

1400 Yards

46:40 min or longer	6½*
46:39—35:00 min	12¾

1400 Yards (Cont.)

34:59—23:20 min	15½
under 23:20 min	21½

1500 Yards

50:00 min or longer	7½*
49:59—37:30 min	14
37:29—25:00 min	17
under 25:00 min	23¼

1600 Yards

53:20 min or longer	8*
53:19—40:00 min	15
39:59—26:40 min	18¼
under 26:40 min	25

1700 Yards

56:40 min or longer	9¾*
56:39—42:30 min	17¼
42:29—28:20 min	20¾
under 28:20 min	28

1800 Yards

1 hr or longer	9½*
59:59—45:00 min	17
44:59—30:00 min	21
under 30:00 min	28½

1900 Yards

1 hr 3:20 min or longer	10*
1 hr 3:19—47:30 min	18½
47:29—31:40 min	22¼
under 31:40 min	30¼

2000 Yards

1 hr 6:40 min or longer	10½
1 hr 6:39—50:00 min	19½
49:59—33:20 min	23½
under 33:20 min	32

ADDITIONAL COMMENTS:

Points calculated on overhand crawl, i.e., 9.0 Kcal per min. Breaststroke is less demanding: 7.0 Kcal per min. Backstroke, a little more: 8.0 Kcal per min. Butterfly, most demanding: 12.0 Kcal per min.

* Exercise of sufficient duration to be of cardiovascular benefit. At this speed, ordinarily no training effect would occur. However, the duration is of such extent that a training effect does begin to occur.

4. POINT VALUE FOR STATIONARY RUNNING

TIME	*60-70 STEPS/MIN	POINTS	*70-80 STEPS/MIN	POINTS	*80-90 STEPS/MIN	POINTS	*90-100 STEPS/MIN	POINTS	*100-110 STEPS/MIN	POINTS
2:30			175-200	¾	200-225	1	225-250	1¼	250-275	1½
5:00	300-350	1¼	350-400	1½	400-450	2	450-500	2½	500-550	3
7:30			525-600	2¼	600-675	3	675-750	3¾	750-825	4½
10:00	600-700	2½	700-800	3	800-900	4	900-1000	5	1000-1100	6
12:30			875-1000	3¾	1000-1125	5	1125-1250	6¼	1250-1375	7½
15:00	900-1050	3¾	1050-1200	4½	1200-1350	6	1350-1500	7½	1500-1650	9
17:30			1225-1400	6¾	1400-1575	8½	1575-1750	10¼	1750-1925	12
20:00	1200-1400	7	1400-1600	8	1600-1800	10	1800-2000	12	2000-2200	14
22:30			1575-1800	9¼	1800-2025	11½	2025-2250	13¾	2250-2475	16
25:00	1500-1750	9¼	1750-2000	10½	2000-2250	13	2250-2500	15½	2500-2750	18
27:30			1925-2200	11¾	2200-2475	14½	2475-2750	17¼	2750-3025	20
30:00	1800-2100	11½	2100-2400	13	2400-2700	16	2700-3000	19	3000-3300	22

* Count only when the left foot hits the floor. Knees must be brought up in front raising the feet at least eight inches from the floor.

5. HANDBALL/BASKETBALL/SQUASH

DURATION *	POINTS	DURATION *	POINTS
10 min	1½	1 hr 10 min	10½
15 min	2¼	1 hr 15 min	11¼
20 min	3	1 hr 20 min	12
25 min	3¾	1 hr 25 min	12¾
30 min	4½	1 hr 30 min	13½
35 min	5¼	1 hr 35 min	14¼
40 min	6	1 hr 40 min	15
45 min	6¾	1 hr 45 min	15¾
50 min	7½	1 hr 50 min	16½
55 min	8¼	1 hr 55 min	17¼
1 hr	9	2 hrs	18
1 hr 5 min	9¾		

* Continuous exercise. Do not count breaks, time-outs, etc.

6. ADDITIONAL EXERCISES

EXERCISE	DURATION	POINTS*	COMMENTS
Badminton	1 game	1½	Singles, players of equal ability,
	2 games	3	and a duration per game of 20
	3 games	4½	minutes.
Fencing	10 min	1	
	20 min	2	
	30 min	3	
Football	30 min	3	Count only the time in which you
	60 min	6	are actively participating.
	90 min	9	
Golf	9 holes	1½	No motorized carts!
	18 holes	3	
Hockey	20 min	3	Count only the time in which you
	40 min	6	are actively participating.
	60 min	9	
	80 min	12	
Lacrosse and	20 min	3	Count only the time in which you
Soccer	40 min	6	are actively partcipating.
	60 min	9	
Rope skip-	5 min	1½	Skip with both feet together or
ping	10 min	3	step over the rope alternating one
	15 min	4½	foot at a time.

*Points based on caloric requirements expressed in the scientific literature.

6. ADDITIONAL EXERCISES (CONTINUED)

EXERCISE	DURATION	POINTS*	COMMENTS
Rowing	6 min	1	2 oars, 20 strokes a minute,
	18 min	4	continuous rowing.
	36 min	8	
Skating	15 min	1	Either ice or roller skating. For
	30 min	2	speed skating triple the point
	60 min	4	value.
Skiing	30 min	3	Water or snow skiing. For cross-
	60 min	6	country snow skiing triple the
	90 min	9	point value.
Tennis	1 set	1½	Singles, players of equal ability,
	2 sets	3	and duration per set of 20 min-
	3 sets	4½	utes.
Volleyball	15 min	1	
	30 min	2	
	60 min	4	
Wrestling	5 min	2	
	10 min	4	
	15 min	6	

* Points based on caloric requirements expressed in the scientific literature.

7. TARGET HEART RATES TO BE USED DURING STRESS TESTING TO DETERMINE THE PRESENCE OR ABSENCE OF HEART DISEASE

AGE (years)	HEART RATE (beats per minute)
under 30	175
30—34	170
35—39	165
40—44	160
45—49	155
50—54	150
55—59	145
60—64	140
65 and up	135

8. DETERMINATION OF THE HEAT STRESS
Wet Bulb Globe Temperature (WBGT) Index *

A. To determine the WBGT index, it is necessary to take readings from (1) a standard thermometer shaded from the sun (2) a black globe thermometer exposed to the sun and prevailing wind and (3) a stationary wet bulb thermometer similarly exposed.

To measure the black globe temperature, obtain a 6-inch hollow copper sphere painted flat black on the outside. Insert a thermometer into the sphere with its bulb at the center. The thermometer is supported by means of a rubber stopper tightly fitting into a brass tube soldered into the sphere. The sphere is supported by two wires or strings and it must be kept dull black by repainting when necessary.

To measure the wet bulb temperature, cover the bulb of a standard laboratory thermometer with a wick (heavy white corset- or shoe-string). Insert the wick into a flask of clean, perferably distilled, water. The mouth of the flask should be about ¾ to 1 inch below the tip of the thermometer bulb and the water level in the flash should be high enough to insure thorough wetting of the wick. The water should be changed daily and the wick washed with soap and water.

B. The WBGT heat stress index is determined as follows:
.7X wet bulb temperature plus .2X black globe temperature plus .1X standard temperature (shade) = WBGT Index

C. How to use the WBGT Index in controlling physical activity.
1. When the WBGT Index exceeds 85° F., only those people who have been exercising in the heat for at least 10 days can continue their workouts.
2. When the WBGT Index exceeds 88° F., only those individuals who have been exercising in the heat for at least 30 days can continue vigorous outdoor workouts.
3. If the WBGT Index exceeds 90° F., it is best for all individuals to stop vigorous outdoor exercise regardless of the state of conditioning or heat acclimatization.

---

* Taken from Air Force Pamphlet 160-1 (25 April 1969), page 9.

METHOD FOR CONSTRUCTING A WBGT INDEX FIELD APPARATUS

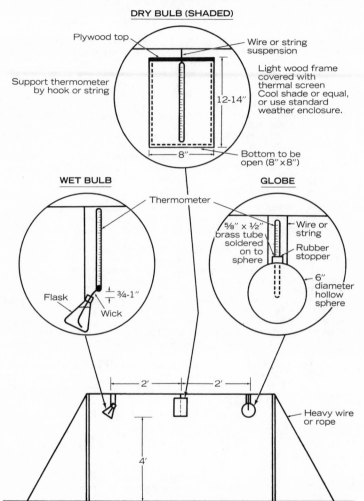

DRY BULB (SHADED)

Plywood top

Wire or string suspension

Support thermometer by hook or string

Light wood frame covered with thermal screen Cool shade or equal, or use standard weather enclosure.

12-14″

8″

Bottom to be open (8″ x 8″)

WET BULB

Thermometer

Flask

¾-1″

Wick

GLOBE

⅝″ x ½″ brass tube soldered on to sphere

Wire or string

Rubber stopper

6″ diameter hollow sphere

2′   2′

Heavy wire or rope

4′

Bibliography

CHAPTER 1

The Texas Poll—Belden Associates—Southland Center, Dallas, Texas, 17 July 1968.

The Coronary Prevention Program For Vermont Communities—Directed by Otto A. Brusis, M.D. Asst. Professor Community Medicine, University of Vermont, Burlington, Vt., April 1969.

Fox, S. M. and Haskell, W. L. "Physical Activity and the Prevention of Coronary Heart Disease." *Bulletin of the New York Academy of Medicine.* Second Series Vol. 44 (No. 8): 950-67, Aug. 1968.

Mitchell, J. H., and Blomqvist, C. G. "Role of Exercise in Prophylaxis Against Coronary Disease." Editorial. *Dallas Medical Journal* Vol. 54: 534-35, November 1968.

Raab, W. "Preventive medical mass reconditioning abroad—Why not in the U.S.A.?" *Ann. Int. Med.* 54:1191, 1961.

Raab, W. R., and Gilman, L. B. "Insurance-Sponsored, Preventive, Cardiac Reconditioning Centers in West Germany." *Amer. J. of Cardiol.* Vol. 13 (No. 5): 670-73, May 1964.

CHAPTER 2

Bevegard, S., Holmgren, A., and Jonsson, B. "Circulatory studies in well-trained athletes at rest and during heavy exercise with special reference to stroke volume and the influence of body position." *Acta Physiol. Scand.* 57:26, 1963.

Cooper, K. H. *Aerobics.* New York: M. Evans & Co. Inc., 1968, pp. 22-30; 56-102.

Cooper, K. H. "Testing and Developing Cardiovascular Fitness Within the United States Air Force." *Journal of Occupational Med.* 10:636–39, November 1968.

Konditionstraning & Konditionstestning. *Fysisk Träning Häfte 1 Chefen For Armen Ao* nr 80: 56, 4/2 1964.

Holmgren, A.; Mossfeldt, F.; Sjöstrand, T.; and Ström G. "Effect of training on work capacity, total hemoglobin, blood volume, heart volume and pulse rate in recumbent and upright positions." *Acta Physiol. Scand.* 50: 72-83, 1960.

Oscai, L. B., Williams, B. T., and Hertig, B. A. "Effect of exercise on blood volume." *Journ. App. Physiol.,* Vol. 24 (No. 5): 622–24, May 1968.

Pyorala, K., Heinonen, A. O., and Karvonen, M. J. "Pulmonary Function in Former Endurance Athletes," *Acta Med. Scand.* Vol. 183; 263–73, 1968.

Saltin, B.; Blomqvist, G.; Mitchell, J. H.; et al. "Response to Exercise After Bed Rest and After Training." *Circulation* 38 (Suppl. 17): 1–78, November 1968.

Wang, Y.; Shepherd, J. T.; Marshall, R. J.; Rowell, L.; and Taylor, H. L. "Cardiac response to exercise in unconditioned young men and in athletes." *Circulation* 24:1064, 1961.

CHAPTER 3

AMA Committee on Exercise and Physical Fitness. "Is Your Patient Fit?" *JAMA* 201: 117–118, (July 10) 1967.

Cooper, K. H. "Guidelines in the Management of the Exercising Patient." *JAMA.* (in press)

"Catch Larry Lewis; He's Only 102" *Fort Smith* (Ark). *Southwest Times-Record.* July 15, 1969.

Grimby, G. and Saltin, B. "Physiological Analysis of Well-trained Middle-aged and Old Athletes." *Acta Med. Scand.* Vol. 179 (fasc 5): 513–526, 1966.

Lester, M.; Sheffield, L. T.; Trammell, P. and Reeves, T. J. "The effect of age and athletic training on the maximal heart rate during muscular exercise." *American Heart Journal* Vol. 76 (No. 3): 370–76, September 1968.

Master, A. M.: "The Master Two-Step Test." *Amer. Heart J.* 75:809–37, June 1963.

CHAPTER 4

Adams, A. "Effect of exercise upon ligament strength." *Res. Quart* 37: 163–67, 1966.

Letter from Coach Thomas L. Bateman III. 30 July 1969. Calvert Hall High School, Towson, Maryland 21204.

Cooper, K. H. "A Means of Assessing Maximal Oxygen Intake," *JAMA* 203: 201–04, 15 January 1968.

Kattus, A. A. Jr.; Hanafee, W. N.; Longmire, W. P. Jr.; McAlpin, R. N.; and Rivin, A. U. "Diagnosis, Medical and Surgical Management of Coronary Insufficiency. *Annals of Internal Medicine* 69:115, July 1968.

"Packers Run to Get Their 2nd Wind." *Milwaukee Journal,* June 29, 1969.

Tipton, C. M., Schild, R. J., and Tomanek, R. J. Influence of physical activity on the strength of knee ligaments in rats. *Amer. J. Physiol.* 212: 783–87, 1967.

Personal communication from Hptn Arthur Zechner, Salzburg, Austria. (27 January 1969).

CHAPTER 5

Air Force Pamphlet 160-4-1. The Etiology, Prevention, Diagnosis and Treatment of Adverse Effects of Heat. 7 August 1957.

Anderson, K. L., Hellström, B., and Eide, R. Strenuous Muscular Exertion in the Polar Climate. *Ergonomics* Vol. 11 (No. 3): 261–74, 1968.

Bowerman, W. From a presentation given to the San Diego Heart Association, San Diego, Calif. 17 June 1968.

Coleman, W. Summer Conditioning Cuts Football Heat Stroke. *Medicine in Sports Newsletter* Vol. 8: No. 4, July 1968.

Hellström, R. and Linroth, K. Physical Working Capacity, Training and Climate. *Acta Med. Scand.* Suppl 472: 207–14, March 11, 1967.

Peter, J., and Wyndham, C. H. Activity of the human eccrine sweat gland during exercise in a hot, humid environment before and after acclimatization. *J. Physiol.* 187: 583–94, 1966.

Stampfer, M.; Epstein, S.; Beiser, G.; Goldstein R.; and Braunwald, E. From a presentation given at the American Heart Association Meeting. "Effect of cold air on peripheral arteries." Bal Harbour, Fla., 24 November 1968.

Strydom, N. B.; Wyndham, C. H.; Williams, C. G.; Morrison, J. F.; Bredell, G. A. G.; Benade, A. J. S.; and Von Rahden, M. Acclimatization to humid heat and the role of physical conditioning. *J. Appl. Physiol.* Vol. 21: 636–42, March 1966.

Taylor, C. L. and Allen, S. C. "Unpublished Report to the National Research Council," 1941.

CHAPTER 6

None

CHAPTER 7

Behling, F. L. (Stress fractures) from an article in *Hospital Tribune,* May 5 1969.

Glick, J. M. and Katch, V. L. Orthopaedic Aspects of Jogging. Presented at the Postgraduate Course on Sports Medicine, July 30, 1969, San Francisco, Calif.

Hoffman, M. S. Jogging and Foot Problems. Letters to the Journal, *JAMA* Vol. 207 (No. 12): 2283–4, March 24, 1969.

Siegel, I. M. Joggers Heel. Letters to the Journal, *JAMA* Vol. 206 (No. 13): 2899, December 23–30, 1968.

CHAPTER 8

Barach, A. L., Bickerman, H. A., and Beck, G. J. Advances in Treatment of Non-Tuberculous Pulmonary Disease. *Bull N. Y. Acad Med* 28:353, 1952.

Campbell, D. E. Influence of several physical activities on serum cholesterol concentrations in young men. *Journal of Lipid Research* Vol. 6: 478–80, 1965.

Carlsson, C., Physician in charge of alcoholics at the mental hospital in Göteborg, Sweden (Lillhagens sjukhus, Hisings-Backa). Communication 13 February 1969. A special report is to be printed in *Quart J.* on Studies of Alcoholism.

Christie, D. Physical Training in Chronic Obstructive Lung Disease. *Brit. Med J* pp 150–151, 20 April 1968.

Frommeyer, W. B. From a Speech given to San Antonio Heart Association, 27 June 1969, San Antonio, Texas.

Golding, L. A. Effects of Physical Training Upon Total Serum Cholesterol Levels. *Rsch Quarterly* Vol. 32 (No. 4): 499, December 1961.

Hellerstein, H. K.; Hornsten, T. R.; Goldbarg, A. N.; Burlando, A. G.; Friedman, E. H.; and Hirsch, E. Z. "The Influence of active conditioning upon coronary atherosclerosis" in *Atherosclerotic Vascular Disease*. Edited by A. N. Brest and J. H. Moyer. New York: Appleton-Century-Crofts, 1967. p 115 (Mood & anxiety changes in response to exercise).

Millman, M.; Grundon, W. G.; Kasch, F.; Wilkerson, B.; and Headley, J. Controlled Exercise in Asthmatic Children. *Annals of Allergy* Vol. 23: 220–25, May 1965.

Paez, P. N.; Phillipson, E. A.; Masangkay, M.; and Sproule, B. J. The Physiologic Basis of Training Patients with Emphysema. *Amer. Review of Respiratory Disease* Vol. 95 (No. 6): 944–53, June 1967.

Pierce, A. K.; Taylor, H. F.; Archer, R. K.; and Miller, W. F. Responses to Exercise Training in Patients wtih Emphysema. *Arch Int. Med* Vol. 113: 78–86, January 1964.

Rochelle, R. H. Blood plasma Cholesterol Changes during a Physical Training Program. *Rsch Quart* Vol. 32 (No. 4): 538, December 1961.

Siegel, W., Blomqvist, G., and Mitchell, J. H. Effects of a Quantitated Physical Training Program on Middle-Aged Sedentary Males. Unpublished report from Southwestern Medical School, Dallas, Texas. (Self image changes in response to exercise.)

CHAPTER 9

Biddulph, L. G. Athletic Achievement and the Personal and Social Adjustment of High School Boys. *Rsch. Quart.* 25 (No. 1), March 1954.

Bier, R. A. How Fit Are Our Youth? *Chicago Medicine* Vol. 71 (No. 19): 731–36, September 14, 1968.

Biörck, G. The Biology of Myocardial Infraction *Circulation* Volume XXXVII: 1071–1085, June 1968.

Brummer, P. Coronary Heart Disease and the Living Standard. *Acta Medica Scandinavica* Vol. 182 (fasc. 4): 523–27, 1967.

Cooper, K. H. A Means of Assessing Maximal Oxygen Intake. *JAMA* 203: 201–204, 15 January 1968.

Doolittle, T. L. and Bigbee, R. The twelve-minute run-walk: A test of cardiorespiratory fitness of adolescent boys. *Rsch. Quart.* 39(3): 491–95, October 1968.

Gallagher, J. R. and Brouha, L. Dynamic Physical Fitness in Adolescence. *Yale Journal of Biology and Medicine* Vol. 15 (No. 5): 657–70, May 1943.

Gendel, E. S. Pregnancy, Fitness, and Sports. *JAMA* Vol. 201 (No. 10): 751–54, September 4, 1967.

Hammerton, M. and Tickner, A. H. Physical Fitness and Skilled Work After Exercise. *Ergonomics* Vol. 11 (No. 1): 41–45, 1968.

Hart, M. E. and Shay, C. T. Relationship Between Physical Fitness and Academic Success. *Rsch. Quart.* 35 (No. 3): 443–45, October 1964.

Rasch, P. J. and Hamby, J. W. Physical Fitness of Women Marines. Vol. XVII (No. 1): January 1967. Bureau of Medicine and Surgery. Navy Dept. Work Unit M.F. 022 01–04–8003.2.

Rose, L. I.; Bradley, E. M.; Kudzma, D. J.; and Cooper, K. H. Changes in Body Composition During Intensive Physical Conditioning (abstract). *Clinical Research* Vol. 17 (No. 2): 393, April 1969.

Walker, A. Coronary Heart Disease and Future Expectation of Life. *Circulation* Vol. XXXVII: 126–31, January 1968.

Weber, R. J. Relationship of Physical Fitness to Success in College and to Personality. *Rsch. Quart.* 24: 471, December 1953.

CHAPTER 10

Gordon, E. E. Energy Cost of Activities in Health and Disease. *AMA Archives of Internal Med* Vol. 101: 702–13, January–June 1958.

Lehmann, G., Arbeitsbedingungen. Praktische Arbeitsphysiologie, Thieme Stuttgart, West Germany, page 154. (Reference on Stairclimbing.) 1953.

Margaria, R.; Cerretelli, P.; Aghemo, P.; and Sassi, G. Energy Cost of Running. *Journ of Applied Physiology* Vol. 18: 367–70, 1963.

CHAPTER 11

Banister, E. W.; Ribisl, P. M.; Porter, G. H.; and Cillo, A. R. The Caloric Cost of Playing Handball. *Rsch. Quart.* 35(3) Part 1: 236–40, October 1964.

"1152 Start, Most Finish" *The Boston Globe,* April 22, 1969.

Bouchard, C.; Hollmann, W.; Venrath, H.; Herkenrath, G.; and Schlussel, H. Minimal Amount of Physical Training for the Prevention of Cardiovascular Diseases. A report from the Dept. of Phys. Ed., Universiteé Laval, Quebec, and Institut fur Kreislaufforschung and Sportmedizin, Köln, Deutschland, June 1968.

Cooper, K. H.; Gey, G. O.; and Bottenberg, R. A. Effects of Cigarette Smoking on Endurance Performance. *JAMA* Vol. 203: 189–92, 15 January 1968.

Doyle, J. T.; Dawber, T. R.; Kannel, W. B.; Kinch, S. H.; and Kahn, H. A. The Relationship of Cigarette Smoking to Coronary Heart Disease. *JAMA* Vol. 190: 886–90, December 7, 1964.

Gey, G. O., Cooper, K. H., and Bottenberg, R. A. Effect of Vitamin C on Endurance Performance and the Incidence, Severity, and Duration of Athletic Injury (A Negative Study). *JAMA* (in press)

Gordon, E. E. Energy Costs of Activities in Health and Disease. *AMA Archives of Internal Medicine* Vol. 101: 702–13, January–June 1958.

Jacobs, E. Smoking Versus Myocardial Infarction: Two Hundred Consecutive Well-Documented Cases. *Military Medicine* Vol. 133: 908–10, 1968.

Karvonen, M. J.; Kentala, E.; and Mustala, O. The Effects of Training on Heart Rate: A Longitudinal Study. *Ann. Med. Exp. Biol. Fenn.,* 35: 307–15, 1957.

MacAlpin, R. N. and Kattus, A. A. Adaptation to Exercise in Angina Pectoris. *Circulation* Volume 33: 233–69, February 1966.

Pollack, M. L., Cureton, T. K., and Greninger, M. S. Effects of frequency of training on working capacity, cardiovascular function, and body composition of adult men. *Medicine and Science in Sports* Vol. 1 (No. 2): 70–74, June 1969.

Roskamm, H. Optimum Patterns of Exercise for Healthy Adults. *Canad. Med. Ass. J.* 96: 895–99, March 25, 1967.

Smith, J. E. and Kidera, G. J. Treamtnt of Angina Pectoris with Exercise Stress. *Aerospace Medicine* Vol. 38 (No. 7): 742–45, July 1967.